The *Essential Clinical Skills for Nurses* series focuses on key clinical skills for nurses and other health professionals. These concise, accessible books assume no prior knowledge and focus on core clinical skills, clearly presenting common clinical procedures and their rationale, together with the essential background theory. Their user-friendly format makes them an indispensable guide to clinical practice for all nurses, especially to student nurses and newly qualified staff.

Other titles in the *Essential Clinical Skills for Nurses* series:

Central Venous Access Devices
Lisa Dougherty
ISBN: 978-1-4051-1952-8

Clinical Assessment and Monitoring in Children
Diana Fergusson
ISBN: 978-1-4051-3338-8

Intravenous Therapy
Theresa Finlay
ISBN: 978-0-6320-6451-9

Respiratory Care
Caia Francis
ISBN: 978-1-4051-1717-3

Care of the Neurological Patient
Helen Iggulden
ISBN: 978-1-4051-1716-6

ECGs for Nurses
Phil Jevon
ISBN: 978-0-6320-5802-0

Monitoring the Critically Ill Patient
Second Edition
Phil Jevon and Beverley Ewens
ISBN: 978-1-4051-4440-7

Treating the Critically Ill Patient
Phil Jevon
ISBN: 978-1-4051-4172-7

Pain Management
Eileen Mann and Eloise Carr
ISBN: 978-1-4051-3071-4

Leg Ulcer Management
Christine Moffatt, Ruth Martin and Rachael Smithdale
ISBN: 978-1-4051-3476-7

Practical Resuscitation
Edited by Pam Moule and John Albarran
ISBN: 978-1-4051-1668-8

Pressure Area Care
Edited by Karen Ousey
ISBN: 978-1-4051-1225-3

Stoma Care
Theresa Porrett and Anthony McGrath
ISBN: 978-1-4051-1407-3

Caring for the Perioperative Patient
Paul Wicker and Joy O'Neill
ISBN: 978-1-4051-2802-5

Infection Prevention and Control

Christine Perry
M.Sc. PG Dip. RN.
Nurse Consultant/Director
Infection Prevention and Control
United Bristol Healthcare Trust
Bristol
UK

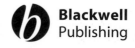

Blackwell
Publishing

Blackwell Publishing editorial offices:
Blackwell Publishing Ltd, 9600 Garsington Road, Oxford OX4 2DQ, UK
Tel: +44 (0)1865 776868
Blackwell Publishing Inc., 350 Main Street, Malden, MA 02148-5020, USA
Tel: +1 781 388 8250
Blackwell Publishing Asia Pty Ltd, 550 Swanston Street, Carlton, Victoria 3053,
Australia
Tel: +61 (0)3 8359 1011

First published 2007 by Blackwell Publishing Ltd

ISBN: 978-1-4051-4038-6

Library of Congress Cataloging-in-Publication Data

Infection prevention and control / edited by Christine Perry.
p. ; cm. – (Essential clinical skills for nurses)
Includes bibliographical references and index.
ISBN-13: 978-1-4051-4038-6 (pbk. : alk. paper)
1. Cross infection–Prevention. 2. Nosocomial infections–
Prevention. 3. Infection–Nursing. 4. Nursing. 5. Hospital buildings–
Sanitation. I. Perry, Christine, MSc. II. Series.
[DNLM: 1. Infection Control–methods. 2. Cross Infection–prevention &
control. 3. Infection–nursing. WC 195 I433 2007]
RA969.I5448 2007
614.4'4–dc22
2007010211

A catalogue record for this title is available from the British Library

Set in 9 on 11 pt Palatino
by SNP Best-set Typesetter Ltd., Hong Kong
Printed and bound in Singapore
by Utopia Press Pte Ltd

The publisher's policy is to use permanent paper from mills that operate a
sustainable forestry policy, and which has been manufactured from pulp
processed using acid-free and elementary chlorine-free practices. Furthermore, the
publisher ensures that the text paper and cover board used have met acceptable
environmental accreditation standards.

For further information on Blackwell Publishing, visit our website:
www.blackwellnursing.com

Contents

List of contributors   vii
Preface   ix
Acknowledgements   x

1   The Function and Structure of Infection Prevention
        and Control Services   1

2   Microbes, Infection and Immunity   13
        Robert C. Spencer

3   Specimen Collection   38

4   Risk Assessment   57

5   Standard Infection Control Principles   66

6   Specific and Common Infections   96

7   Infection Prevention in Urinary Catheter Care   140
        Lauren Tew

8   Infection Prevention in Intravascular Therapy   154
        Carly Hall

9   Infection Prevention in Nutritional Care   177

10 Infection Prevention in Wound Management   187

11 Control of Infection in Paediatric Settings   197

12 Peri-operative Care Settings   220

13 Specialist Care Settings   239

14 The Isolated Patient   254

Contents

15 The Immunocompromised Patient   267

16 Decontamination   275

Index   288

Contributors

Dr Carly Hall Ph.D. B.Sc.(Hons) RN
Senior Infection Control Nurse
United Bristol Healthcare Trust
Bristol
UK

Dr Robert C. Spencer MB BS M.Sc. FRCPath FRCP(G) Hon
   DipHIC
Consultant Microbiologist
Health Protection Agency
Bristol
UK
and Chairman Hospital Infection Society

Lauren Tew B.Sc.(Hons) PGDip(HE) RNT RN
Infection Control Clinical Consultant
Bristol
UK

Preface

The early years of the twenty-first century have seen the prevention and control of healthcare associated infections become more high profile than ever before. It is the duty of all healthcare staff to practice in a way that prevents risk of infection to themselves and to the patients in their care. The purpose of this book is to provide nurses and other healthcare staff with knowledge and skills to help them practice safely. Although infection prevention is important in all the environments in which patients receive health and social care, patients in hospital have an increased risk of infection due to their contact with other people with infections and the procedures that they undergo during their hospitalisation. Whilst principles of infection prevention remain the same wherever patients receive care, this book concentrates predominantly on prevention of infection in acute hospital care. It is intended for use as an aide-memoire and whereas the principles of infection prevention remain the same, individual hospital policies and procedures should always be referred to.

Christine Perry
Nurse Consultant Infection Prevention and Control
United Bristol Healthcare Trust

Acknowledgements

The editor is grateful to:

- Joanna Davies, Senior Infection Control Nurse, United Bristol Healthcare Trust, for her help with writing Chapter 12
- Stephanie Carroll, Infection Control Sister, United Bristol Healthcare Trust, for her help with writing Chapter 5
- Michelle Lindsay, Infection Control Sister, United Bristol Healthcare Trust, for her help with writing Chapter 3
- Angela Cherrington, Infection Control Sister, United Bristol Healthcare Trust, for her help with writing Chapter 6
- Dr J.P. Leeming, Clinical Scientist, Health Protection Agency, Bristol, for providing photography

The Function and Structure of Infection Prevention and Control Services

1

INTRODUCTION

Prevention and control of infection is important for legal, professional and economical reasons. Within any healthcare organisation infection prevention and control operates at practical, managerial and strategic levels. This chapter outlines the development of infection prevention and control services, national and legal requirements, the structure and function of infection control services and the link to clinical risk management and governance.

LEARNING OBJECTIVES

By the end of this chapter you will be able to:

❑ Detail significant events that have shaped infection prevention and control in UK hospitals
❑ Describe the organisation of infection prevention and control services
❑ Identify the key policies and initiatives relevant to infection prevention and control
❑ Identify the healthcare workers' role in infection prevention

THE HISTORICAL PERSPECTIVE

The importance of infection prevention has been recognised as far back as biblical times and is still important in the early years of the twenty-first century. Leper colonies were instituted to separate infected people from the rest of the population and the 'unclean' bell was used to warn people to stay away. During the plague of 1665, bodies were collected at night to minimise contact with healthy people. Although very primitive in design, the plague doctor wore protective clothing in the form of a gown, mask and gloves. In the early 1800s, the Hungarian obstetrician, Semelweiss, noted that more mothers were dying from infections after childbirth when doctors and medical students delivered the babies than when they were delivered by midwives. In his observations he noted that the medical staff were coming straight from the post-mortem room to the delivery room without washing their hands and he deduced that this was the route of cross infection. He instituted the procedure of hand washing with chloride of lime and dropped the infection and death rate almost instantaneously.

Florence Nightingale is probably the first nurse on record to recognise the importance of prevention of infection. From her observations of the hospital at Scutari during the Crimean War, she noted that more soldiers were dying from infections than from their war injuries. Although she did not believe in the presence of micro-organisms, she recognised that placing together a large number of sick people in an area with inadequate space, light and ventilation was contributing to the spread of infection. She introduced hygiene protocols and, through collecting the appropriate data, demonstrated a reduction in rates of infection. Some of the principles she applied are still of relevance today and she believed that if proper sanitary precautions were applied, it was possible to treat patients with infectious diseases in wards without danger to other patients. This approach is still echoed today in the principles of universal or standard precautions. The advent of penicillin in the 1940s led to a new era in infection management. For the first time, infections could be treated and deaths due to infection avoided. Prevention of infection became less important now that treatment was available.

In the late 1950s a pandemic of infections due to *Staphylococcus aureus* drove hospitals to reconsider infection prevention measures. In 1959 the first recorded appointment of an infection control nurse was made at Torquay Hospital (Worsley, 1988). At that time, the microbiologist was based at Exeter, 30 miles away, and could not visit Torquay on a daily basis. The infection control sister was responsible for supervision of infection prevention activities and advising on individual patient management. The overall management of infection prevention was strengthened and every hospital in England was required to have an infection control committee and an infection control officer, who was usually a doctor. Infection prevention and control services slowly developed in the ensuing years, but in the 1980s the advent of the human immunodeficiency virus (HIV) and acquired immune deficiency syndrome (AIDS) led to a renewed interest and approach to infection prevention. The risk of infection for health-care staff, and the fact that patients could have these infections without displaying symptoms led to a shift away from infection precautions depending on a patient's infection status to assuming any patient could have an infection and taking precautions for all patients. In the late 1980s a significant event in the UK led to further strengthening of infection control services. An outbreak of salmonella food poisoning at Stanley Royd Hospital in Yorkshire led to the deaths of several patients. This prompted the Department of Health to issue instructions that all health districts should appoint an infection control nurse and develop clear contingency plans for managing outbreaks of infections (DHSS, 1988).

The early 1990s saw a resurgence of *Staphylococcus aureus* infections, but this time with epidemic strains of the bacteria that were meticillin resistant. Hospitals again came under scrutiny over their infection prevention and control structures. A report by the National Audit Office on infection prevention in English and Welsh Hospitals, undertaken in 1998, suggested that hospital acquired infections were costing £1 billion and were contributing to up to 5000 deaths per year in the UK (National Audit Office, 2000). The devolved healthcare administrations throughout the UK each addressed this individually, but in similar ways, with the development of strategies to prevent healthcare associated infection. Reporting of important healthcare associated infections became compulsory for most of the countries in the UK, with results being made publicly available. Although hospitals had some legal obligations for infection prevention related to health and safety, it became law in England for hospitals to abide by a hygiene code of practice in 2006 (DoH, 2006). This has underlined the importance of adherence to good infection prevention and control practice at clinical level, as well as having the appropriate structures in place to monitor and report infections, besides acting on infection outbreaks and reducing risk within all hospitals.

WHY INFECTION PREVENTION AND CONTROL IS IMPORTANT

The Health and Safety at Work Act (HSE, 2003) requires organisations to take steps to protect staff and visitors on their premises from hazards and risks. Within a hospital, this includes risk of infection and applies to staff, patients and visitors. The Control of Substances Hazardous to Health Regulations (HSE, 1999) also applies to prevention of infection, as micro-organisms are considered to be hazardous substances. Under these regulations it is a requirement that healthcare organisations:

(1) Assess the risk of contact with a hazardous substance.
(2) Remove the hazardous substance where possible.
(3) If it is not possible to remove the substance then prevent contact.
(4) If it is not possible to prevent contact then provide employees with protective clothing.

In addition to health and safety law, in England the Health Act 2006 (DoH, 2006) requires NHS trusts to provide care in accordance with the code. The code sets out statutory requirements in the following areas:

- Management
- Accountability
- Assurance arrangements
- Clinical care protocols
- Decontamination of equipment
- Surveillance
- Occupational health
- Education and training

The Healthcare Commission, who can issue an improvement notice if non-compliance is evident, assesses hospitals in England for their compliance to this code. If NHS trusts fail to act on this, sanctions can be taken against trust chief executives and boards through strategic health authorities, or foundation trusts through monitor.

As well as the legal necessity to prevent infections, healthcare staff have a professional responsibility to patients in their care.

Under the *Nursing Code of Conduct* (NMC, 2004), nurses are required to identify and minimise risk to patients and clients; this will include infection control risks. A similar requirement is also placed on medical staff, through the British Medical Association and on other health professionals through the Health Professions Council. It is also usual for NHS trusts to place an expectation of staff that they operate within trust policies and procedures, and this will generally include infection control policies and procedures.

From an economic perspective, prevention of infection is important for financial and resource management. The average additional cost of each healthcare associated infection is in excess of £3154 (Plowman *et al.*, 2000), with length of patient stay extended by on average 11 days. With certain infections the additional length of stay can be even greater, for example 21 days on average for patients with *Clostridium difficile* (Wilcox *et al.*, 1996). Of prime importance in healthcare is the patient's experience and outcome. For the patient, a healthcare associated infection can lead to increased pain, further investigations or surgery, additional drugs and treatments and, in extreme circumstances, death. Infections are still associated with a stigma of uncleanliness and fear of passing them from patients to relatives and carers. For patients who need to be placed in single rooms to prevent spread of infection, there are also the implications of isolation both physically and mentally.

THE EXTENT OF HOSPITAL INFECTIONS

Many patients admitted to hospital will already have an infection apparent or incubating. It is generally accepted that where patients develop signs and symptoms of infection within 48 hours of admission it is more likely that they acquired the infection before their admission to hospital. Hospital admission carries a risk of infection due to patients being exposed to other patients with infections, as well as risks associated with procedures undertaken during their hospitalisation. The presence of an invasive device, such as a peripheral intravenous cannula, increases the risk of infection and death seven-fold (Glynn *et al.*, 1997). Identifying levels of hospital acquired infection can be done in a number of ways, through both audit and surveillance. The different types of surveillance activities used in acute hospital care are outlined below in Box 1.1.

The most recent survey of hospital acquired infection in the UK and Ireland found an overall prevalence rate of 7.6% (Hospital Infection Society, 2006). The most common infections identified were gastro-intestinal tract and urinary tract (see Figure 1.1).

Box 1.1 Surveillance definitions.

Incidence survey The number of cases of infection that occur in a cohort of patients over a time period. For example, all patients who undergo cardiac bypass surgery over a three-month period are surveyed for surgical wound infection. The number that acquire an infection is the incidence of infection.

Prevalence survey The number of cases of infection in a cohort of patients surveyed over a defined period of time. For example, all patients in a hospital are surveyed for presence of urinary tract infection on a given day. The number of patients who have evidence of infection on that day is the prevalence of infection.

Targeted surveillance The surveillance of specific infections in a defined patient population. For example, the surveillance of urinary tract infection in patients undergoing gynaecological surgery.

Alert organisms surveillance The surveillance of patients who have evidence of specific infections that are considered important in hospital infection control; these are usually identified from laboratory reports, for example the number of patients who are meticillin resistant *Staphylococcus aureus* positive in a hospital over the previous month.

Prospective surveillance The surveillance of infection in patients who are monitored during their hospital stay. For example, patients undergoing hip prosthesis surgery are observed daily during admission, for signs and symptoms of infection.

Retrospective surveillance The surveillance of infection in patients by follow up after the event of hospitalisation. For example, the clinical records of patients who have been on an intensive care unit for the preceding three months are reviewed for signs and symptoms of pneumonia.

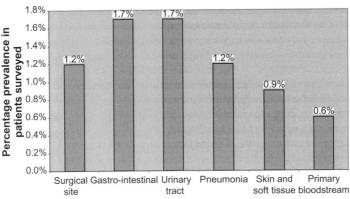

Figure **1.1** Prevalence of hospital acquired infections (Hospital Infection Society, 2006).

Across the UK, reporting of important hospital infections is necessary, for example bacteraemia due to MRSA. This helps to direct national infection control policy and actions. Infection rates for trusts are also generally made available publicly.

INFECTION CONTROL STRUCTURES AND ROLES

Within NHS organisations, the chief executive usually has overall responsibility for infection prevention and control. A board director is also generally allocated as a lead in this area. Between them, they are responsible for ensuring that the appropriate infection control structures and activities are in place. More recently, health departments in the UK have also advised the designation of a key clinician or manager to take responsibility for the delivery of infection control activities. In Wales there must be a designated lead within local management teams. Scotland requires a nurse consultant in infection control in every health board. Northern Ireland requires its hospitals to have a designated infection control lead. This is also required in England, with a director of infection prevention and control designated in every NHS organisation. These people generally have a role in overseeing the work and activities of the infection control team and are an integral member of clinical risk and governance teams.

The infection control doctor is generally a microbiologist, but may be a physician with an interest in infection control. They are responsible for providing specialist microbiological advice to a trust and take an active role in day-to-day infection prevention and management issues. The role of the infection control nurse can be diverse, depending on their position in the trust, but there are core elements to this role.

Core elements of the infection control nurse role

- Education and training
- Clinical advice in support of staff and patients
- Policy development and implementation
- Audit and service improvement
- Surveillance
- Investigation and management of infection outbreaks
- Advice for purchasing and contracting
- Occupational health advice
- Risk assessment and management (Perry, 2005)

Modern matrons were introduced back into the NHS in 2001 (NHSE, 2001). In collaboration with the infection control nurses they have a responsibility for clinical standards and practice related to infection prevention. Within the charter attached to this role the infection control aspects are:

- Tackling standards of cleanliness
- Implementation of national evidence based principles for practice

Many trusts have introduced an infection control link nurse system to support the implementation of infection control at local level (National Audit Office, 2004). They do not undertake the full role of an infection control nurse but they undertake defined activities in their area. The roles often assigned to infection control link nurses are outlined below.

Box 1.2 Other services that support NHS organisations in delivery of safe patient care.

Occupational health departments assess staff for fitness to work (e.g. ensuring catering staff are not carriers of food borne infections), contact tracing and testing of staff who have been exposed to an infectious disease (e.g. chickenpox).

Estates/facilities departments maintain a clean environment, dispose of waste, provide clean linen.

Sterile services departments reprocess surgical instruments and provide sterile procedure packs.

Catering departments supply food that is safe to eat and ensure food preparation areas meet legal requirements.

Pharmacists advise on antibiotic prescribing and monitor use of antibiotics.

All healthcare staff have a responsibility to comply with infection control policies and procedures as set by their employers and to practice in a manner that minimises risks of infection.

Role of infection control link nurses

- To assist in the implementation of infection control policies, guidelines and standards at clinical level
- To act as a communication link between the infection control team and clinical area
- In liaison with the infection control team, to act as a resource person concerning infection control related problems (e.g. isolation, decontamination of equipment)
- To participate in infection control audit
- To contribute to the writing and updating of infection control policies, guidelines and standards
- To participate in the education of staff and patients in infection control related matters
- To bring to the attention of the infection control team outbreaks of infection or infection control related problems in clinical areas

- To bring to the attention of the infection control team practice developments to enable sharing of good practice
- To take every opportunity to extend and update personal knowledge of infection control
- To act as an information resource to assist in ensuring the availability of resources to support infection control practice at clinical level

NHS trusts will generally have an infection control committee that is made up of representatives from the groups mentioned above, together with managerial and clinical input. This committee will monitor the infection prevention and control activities, and receive reports on infection control surveillance and audit programmes, as well as infection outbreaks. It is the role of this committee to advise the chief executive and trust board of infection control risks as well as actions needed to prevent outbreaks of infection.

INFECTION CONTROL AND GOVERNANCE

Prevention of infection is a patient safety issue as well as an indicator of quality of care. Serious outbreaks and incidences of infection, or serious breaches in infection prevention practice, should be reported through a trust's incident reporting procedure. An example of this would be the use of surgical instruments that had not been adequately decontaminated between use. This type of report will usually prompt an investigation leading to corrective action. National bodies, such as the National Patient Safety Agency and the Medicines and Healthcare Products Regulatory Agency collate reports of these types of incidents from trusts and may then issue warning notices to NHS organisations. Governance structures within NHS trusts will generally monitor infection control incidents, complaints and risk assessments. They may also receive reports of infection control audits and surveillance activities. Through these governance processes, NHS trusts are able to provide assurances to the public and Government bodies that they are taking actions to reduce infection risks for staff, visitors and patients. Key components of clinical governance in the NHS include clinical effectiveness, risk management, patient experience and resource effectiveness (Pratt *et al.*, 2002). Clinical audit is a useful process for demonstrating the effectiveness, patient experience and effective management of risk. Infection control audit has been demonstrated to be a valuable tool in assessing the effectiveness of staff training, identifying areas where practice improvements are needed and in monitoring the implementation of infection control policies (Millward *et al.*, 1993). Infection control audit tools that are suitable for use by non-infection control nurses are available (Infection Control Nurses Association, 2004).

EXERCISE

- Find out the latest rate of MRSA bloodstream infection for your nearest NHS hospital on the Internet. If you cannot locate it on the Internet ask your infection control nurse to direct you.
- Locate the infection control policy/manual for your hospital, and from that identify who your infection control team are and how to contact them.

SUMMARY
Prevention of hospital infection requires a multi-faceted approach, including strategic management of a hospital's infection control programme as well as implementation of good infection control practice during clinical care. All healthcare workers have a role to play in prevention of infection in compliance with local policies and procedures. The infection control team plays a key role in a hospital's infection prevention programme; they are often supported in this by infection control link nurses in clinical wards and departments. Hospital governance structures are important in the monitoring and addressing of infection control related risks. Audit of infection control practice is a useful tool in identifying areas where improvements in practice may be needed.

REFERENCES
Department of Health (2006) *The Health Act 2006: Code of Practice for the Prevention and Control of Health Care Associated Infection*. Department of Health, London.
Department of Health and Social Security (1988) *Hospital Infection Control: Guidance on the Control of Infection in Hospitals Prepared by*

the Joint DHSS/PHLS Hospital Infection Working Group. Department of Health and Social Security, London.

Glynn, A., Ward, V., Wilson, J. *et al.* (1997) *Hospital Acquired Infection: Surveillance, Policies and Practice.* Public Health Laboratory Service, London.

Health and Safety Executive (1999) *Control of Substances Hazardous to Health (COSHH) (Amendments) Act.* Health and Safety Executive, London.

Health and Safety Executive (2003) *Health and Safety Regulation . . . a Short Guide.* Health and Safety Executive, London.

Hospital Infection Society (2006) Press release for: *The Third Prevalence Survey of Healthcare Associated Infections in Acute Hospitals.* Available at: http://www.his.org.uk/_db/_documents/Press_information. doc (accessed 20 November 2006).

Infection Control Nurses Association (2004) *Audit Tools for Monitoring Infection Control Standards.* Available from: www.icna.co.uk (accessed 20 November 2006).

Millward, S., Barnett, J. and Thomlinson, D.A. (1993) A clinical infection control audit programme: evaluation of an audit used by infection control nurses to monitor standards and assess effectiveness of staff training. *Journal of Hospital Infection*, **24**, 219–232.

National Audit Office (2000) *The Management and Control of Hospital Acquired Infection in Acute NHS Trusts in England.* The Stationery Office, London.

National Audit Office (2004) *Improving Patient Care by Reducing the Risk of Hospital Acquired Infection: a Progress Report.* The Stationery Office, London.

NHS Executive (2001) *Implementing the NHS Plan – Modern Matrons: Strengthening the Role of Ward Sisters and Introducing Senior Sisters.* Health Service Circular 2001/010. NHS Executive, London.

Nursing and Midwifery Council (2004) *The NMC Code of Professional Conduct: Standards for Conduct, Performance and Ethics.* Available at: http://www.nmc-uk.org/aDisplayDocument.aspx?DocumentID =201 (accessed 20 November 2006).

Perry, C.M. (2005) The infection control nurse in England: past, present, future. *British Journal of Infection Control*, **6** (5), 18–21.

Plowman, R., Graves, N., Griffin, M. *et al.* (2000) *Socio-economic Burden of Hospital Acquired Infection.* Department of Health, London.

Pratt, R., Morgan, S., Hughes, J. *et al.* (2002) Healthcare governance and the modernisation of the NHS: infection prevention and control. *British Journal of Infection Control*, **3** (5), 16–25.

Wilcox, M.H., Cunniffe, J.G., Trundle, C. and Redpath, C. (1996) Financial burden of hospital acquired *Clostridium difficile* infection. *Journal of Hospital Infection*, **34**, 23–30.

Worsley M.A. (1988) The role of the infection control nurse. *Journal of Hospital Infection*, **11** (suppl. A), 400–405.

Microbes, Infection and Immunity

2

Robert C. Spencer

INTRODUCTION

The prevention of hospital infection requires an understanding of how micro-organisms cause infection and spread in a hospital environment. This chapter covers basic aspects of microbiology, the infection process, immunity and the transmission of infection.

LEARNING OBJECTIVES

By the end of this chapter you will be able to:

❏ Describe the structure, physiology and reproduction of medically important micro-organisms
❏ Describe the infection process and the resulting immune response
❏ Identify groups of antimicrobial agents (antibiotics) and their activity against micro-organisms
❏ Describe the processes of antibiotic resistance
❏ State the routes by which micro-organisms are transmitted in a hospital environment

Micro-organisms are found everywhere in nature and are believed to have been the first life form on the planet. Not all micro-organisms are harmful; in the body they can serve useful functions, for example bacteria in the gut can aid digestion through the production of vitamin K and on the skin aid in preventing colonisation by pathogenic bacteria, such as *Staphylococcus aureus*. The study of micro-organisms is known as microbiology. The first micro-organisms to be seen were in the 1670s, by the

Dutch scientist Anthony Van Leeuwenhoek using a crude microscope. Today the study of micro-organisms is still undertaken using conventional microscopes, but through scientific developments, more advanced techniques are used to detect and identify micro-organisms.

BACTERIAL CELLS

Bacteria are prokaryotic cells; they are single celled organisms, enclosed by a membrane rather than a cell wall. They can only be seen under a microscope and range in size from 0.5 to 1 micrometre. Figure 2.1 shows a simplified diagrammatic structure of a bacterial cell.

Cell wall   This is made up of a network of carbohydrates and amino acids called peptidoglycan. The exact make-up of the cell wall varies between different bacteria. The make-up of the cell wall is used to help identify the bacterial species. Gram staining is a process used in the laboratory to determine the type of cell wall. The bacterial cell is coloured using a purple staining agent and then a pink staining agent is applied. If the purple stain is replaced by the pink, then the bacterium is Gram negative; if the

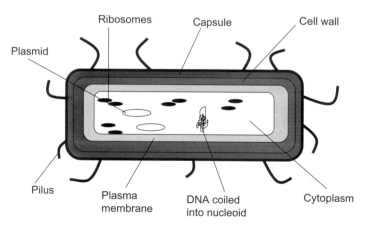

Figure 2.1 Simplified structure of a bacterial cell.

stain remains purple, it is Gram positive. Gram positive bacteria have a cell wall that is composed almost entirely of peptidoglycan. Gram negative bacteria have a cell wall that is a layer of peptidoglycan sandwiched between two membranes. The outer membrane may possess some endotoxins, which can act against the host defences of the patient. The function of the cell wall is to contain the contents of the cell.

Capsule   The capsule is a layer of gelatinous material. Its function is to protect the cell against attack by white blood cells. The capsule helps some bacteria to adhere to surfaces such as teeth and prosthetic devices. This is not present on all bacterial cells.

Plasma membrane   This is a thin cell membrane that encloses the cytoplasm of the cell. The membrane acts as a filter controlling what can enter and exit the cell.

Ribosomes   These are the 'power houses' of the bacterial cell. It is here that amino acids are assembled into proteins.

Cytoplasm   This is where the biochemical reactions of the bacterial cell take place. Food materials, such as glycogen are also stored here.

Nucleus   This contains the genetic material of the cell in the form of deoxyribonucleic acid (DNA). Bacterial cells have only one chromosome.

Plasmid   This is an additional fragment of DNA outside the chromosome, which often carries genetic information regarding antibiotic resistance.

Flagellae   Some bacterial cells have flagellae which are long filaments extending from the surface of the cell. Cells may have as few as one or as many as twenty. Their purpose is motility.

Pili   are shorter and thinner than flagellae and there may be hundreds attached to one cell. Their purpose is adherence to host cells, for example intestinal cells, and other bacteria; they also play a role in transmission of antibiotic resistance from one bacterial cell to another.

Bacteria are classified according to their Gram staining properties: Gram negative or positive. Some bacteria cannot be stained using the Gram method; for example mycobacterium, the causative agent of tuberculosis, which have a waxy coating. A Ziehl-Nielsen or alcohol–acid fast (AAFB) stain is used for identification of these bacteria. The shape of bacteria is also used in their classification.

Cocci are round in shape. They may be arranged in pairs (diplococci), in chains (streptococci) or in clumps like grapes (staphylococci).

Bacilli are rod or cylindrical shaped. They are generally straight, but may be slightly curved (*Escherichia coli, Klebsiella* spp.).

Vibrios are curved rod shaped (*Vibrio cholerae* – the agent that causes cholera).

Spirochaetes are corkscrew like spirals (*Treponema pallidum* – the agent that causes syphilis).

When referring to bacteria by name, two names are generally used: the *genus* (the group of bacteria to which it belongs), for example *Staphylococcus*, and the specific *species* it belongs to within that group, for example *Staphylococcus aureus* or *Staphylococcus epidermidis*.

For bacterial cells to grow and reproduce they have certain requirements:

Water is essential, and most bacteria will die in its absence. Gram negative bacteria in particular will thrive in damp environments.

Temperature Micro-organisms that cause infection in humans generally require temperatures around 37°C; however, some bacteria can multiply at low temperatures, for example listeria at 5°C. Low temperatures will not kill bacteria but can stop replication. High temperatures will destroy bacteria.

Oxygen Bacteria that only reproduce in the presence of oxygen are referred to as *aerobic*. Those that only reproduce in the absence of oxygen are *anaerobic*. Many micro-organisms are able to reproduce either in the absence or presence of oxygen and are referred to as facultative.

pH Most bacteria prefer a neutral solution but some can survive in very acidic or alkaline environments.

Nutrients Bacteria require an energy source, which they obtain from the breakdown of organic carbon containing compounds. They all require a carbon source, which can come from organic compounds such as glucose, but sometimes comes from the atmosphere in the form of carbon dioxide. Nitrogen is needed for the cell structures, such as protein. Some require inorganic ions such as sodium and potassium and trace elements, including iron or zinc to make enzymes.

Bacterial reproduction is by binary fission (Figure 2.2). When the cell has grown to a specific size, the single chromosome divides into two identical chromosomes. The cell wall and membrane grow inwards forming a new cell wall across the cell. Eventually this splits the cytoplasm into two cells, each with a chromosome. Often the two cells do not completely separate but they remain together as clumps, chains or in pairs. Bacteria do

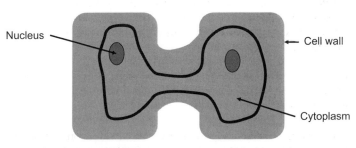

Nucleus

Cell wall

Cytoplasm

The chromosome replicates, a new cell wall forms and divides the original cell into two.

Figure 2.2 Bacterial reproduction by binary fission.

Table 2.1 Characteristics of some medically important bacteria.

Genus and species	Shape	Gram staining	Motility	Oxygen requirement	Spore forming
Staphylococcus aureus	Cocci	Positive	Non-motile	Aerobic	No
Streptococcus pyogenes	Cocci	Positive	Non-motile	Aerobic	No
Escherechia coli	Bacilli	Negative	Motile	Facultative anaerobe	No
Pseudomonas aeruginosa	Bacilli	Negative	Motile	Aerobic	No
Clostridium difficile	Bacilli	Positive	Motile	Anaerobic	Yes

not need living host cells in which to grow and reproduce. Some bacteria have the ability to undergo a resting phase where they survive adverse conditions for extended periods, sometimes for many years. Some bacteria, when faced with adverse conditions, have the ability to form spores, which can, for example, resist drying and persist for years. Examples of these include the bacteria that cause anthrax and gas gangrene. Bacterial spores are more resistant than normal bacteria to heat, drying and disinfection. Given the right conditions they will germinate and start the bacterial growth and reproduction process. Table 2.1 details the characteristics of some of the medically important bacteria.

Rickettsiae and chlamydia possess some of the characteristics of bacteria in that they are prokaryotic cells and reproduce by binary fission, but their genetic material contains both DNA and ribonucleic acid (RNA). They are smaller than bacteria, being of diameter 0.25–0.5 micrometres and only reproduce in a living host cell.

VIRUSES

Viruses cannot be seen using a conventional microscope and require an electron microscope to visualise them, being of size 30 nanometres to 400 nanometres. Figure 2.3 shows a simplified diagrammatic structure of a virus particle.

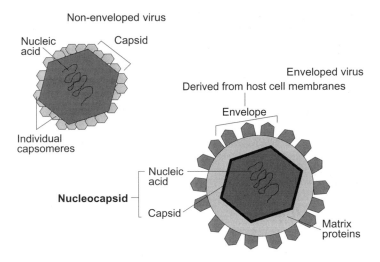

Figure 2.3 Diagrammatic representation of a virus particle.

Virion This is the complete virus particle, consisting of genetic material surrounded by a protective protein coat.

Genome This is the virus nucleic acid and can be either RNA or DNA in single or double strands.

Capsid This is the protein coat around the virion and is composed of subunits called capsomeres.

Nucleocapsid is the combination of nucleic acid and the capsid.

Enveloped viruses have a covering of lipids and proteins that are largely derived from the outer membrane of host reproduction cells. Many virus particles are enveloped, for example influenza.

Non-enveloped or **naked** viruses do not have an envelope. They are more resistant to disinfection and survive better outside a host cell than enveloped viruses, for example hepatitis B.

Glycoproteins These are projections on the surface of some virus particles, for example measles and influenza, that are seen on electron microscopy as well defined spikes.

Viruses are classified according to their size, their nucleid acid (RNA or DNA), the presence or absence of an envelope, their molecular weight and their shape and symmetry.

Isocahedral viruses are regular polyhedrons with 20 triangular faces and 12 corners.

Helical viruses have a herringbone like appearance.

Complex viruses do not conform to either of the above and can be ovoid or brick shaped.

Viruses reproduce strictly inside living host cells. Figure 2.4 is a diagrammatic representation of the process of viral replication. A circulating virus enters the body and then attaches to specific receptors on a host cells. If these receptors are not present then infection will not occur. Once attached, the virus enters or penetrates the host cell (*penetration*). With enveloped viruses this is through fusion with the host cell membrane; with naked viruses this is through direct penetration of the cell membrane. Once inside the host cell, cellular enzymes remove the capsid (*uncoating*) to expose the genome. Messenger RNA is then made which takes the genetic material from the virus particle into the cytoplasm of the host cell, from which new viral proteins to make new capsids and viral nucleic acid are made (*replication*). When these protein coats have been made, they move from the cytoplasm of the host cell into the nucleus, where they combine with the virus DNA (*assembly*). Once new virions are assembled, they are then released from the host cell. Enveloped viruses bud out through the host cell membrane. It is the host cell membrane that then gives them their coating. This form of release does not always cause the host cell to die, therefore, the host cell can continue to manufacture and release more virus particles for some time. Non-enveloped viruses are released from the host cell by a process called cytolysis. This leads to the leaking out of the cell contents and eventually death of the host cell.

Table 2.2 details some of the medically important viruses.

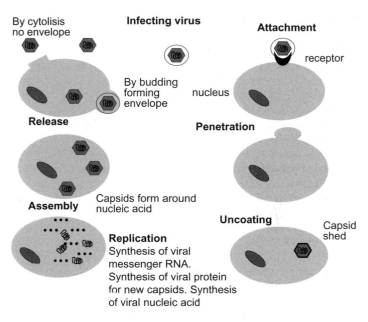

Figure 2.4 Viral replication.

Table 2.2 Some medically important viruses.

Infection group	Causative viruses
Respiratory	Respiratory syncytial virus Influenza SARS – severe acute respiratory syndrome
Skin	Herpes simplex Varicella zoster
Gastro-intestinal	Norovirus Rotavirus

FUNGI

Fungi are eukaryotic cells with a membrane enclosing the cell contents as opposed to a cell wall. They can be divided into three groups:

Table 2.3 Some medically important fungi.

Infection group	Fungi
Cutaneous	Candida, dermatophytes
Genito-urinary	Candida
Invasion	Aspergillus

- **Moulds**, which are filamentous organisms that reproduce by means of spore production, for example *Aspergillus fumigatus*.
- **Yeasts**, which are unicellular and reproduce by a budding process or binary fission, for example *Cryptococcus neoformans*.
- **Dimorphic fungi** Fungal infections are referred to as mycoses and most of the fungi that cause infection in humans are moulds. Superficial mycoses are infections of the skin, nails, hair and mucous membranes. Examples of superficial mycoses in humans are ringworm and *Candida albicans*. Subcutaneous mycoses affect the skin, fascia bone and subcutaneous tissues. Subcutaneous mycoses generally only occur in tropical and subtropical climates. Systemic mycoses are deep-seated infections that generally occur as a result of inhaled fungal spores. In immunocompromised patients there are a number of fungi that can cause systemic mycoses including *Aspergillus* and *Candida*. Table 2.3 details some medically important fungi.

PROTOZOA
Protozoa are large single-celled eukaryotic organisms. They can be divided into four groups:

- **Sporozoa**, of which malaria (*Plasmodium*) is the commonest life-threatening infection
- **Amoeba**, of which *Entamoeba histolytica* is the most important in human disease, causing amoebic dysentery, characterised by bloody diarrhoea
- **Flagellates**, of which *Giardia lamblia* causes diarrhoea

- **Other pathogenic species** that are uncommon causes of human disease in the UK, for example *Balantidium coli*, which causes dysentery

LABORATORY DETECTION METHODS

Identification of micro-organisms in the laboratory can be a complex process involving a number of tests and techniques. The following methods are commonly used for the purpose of detecting micro-organisms and identifying their genus and species (Greenwood *et al.*, 2002).

Culturing is carried out by inoculating specimens onto agar (a derivative of seaweed) jelly that contains a growth medium. As different bacteria have different growth requirements, when a sample, for example a wound swab, is received in the laboratory it will be plated onto a number of different types of agar to ensure that any micro-organisms that may be present are given the optimum conditions in which to grow. Figure 2.5 shows *Staphylococcus aureus* growing on a blood agar plate. Once the specimen has been inoculated onto the agar plate it is incubated at body temperature for a specified time. Most bacteria grow overnight; strains such as the anaerobic bacteria require incubation for 48 to 72 hours to ensure maximal growth. The way in which micro-organisms grow on the agar plate gives an indication of what type of bacteria may be present. Micro-organisms that have grown on the plate can be examined under a microscope and Gram stained.

Microscopy is the examination of micro-organisms under a microscope. Conventional microscopes can be used for bacterial, fungal and protozoal detection, but due to their small size, virus detection requires a high powered electron microscope.

Biochemical reactions These tests examine the ability of cultured micro-organisms to produce end-products. Commercially manufactured test kits are generally used for this purpose and can be used to identify groups of micro-organisms that include staphylococci and streptococci.

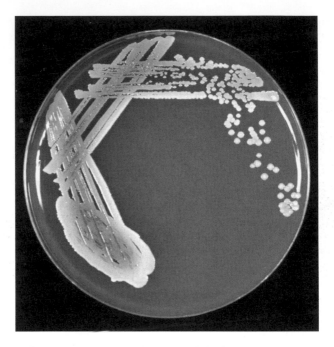

Figure 2.5 *Staphylococcus aureus* growing on a blood agar plate (picture courtesy of Dr J.P. Leeming).

Sensitivity testing is carried out on potentially pathogenic cultured bacteria. A solution containing the cultured bacteria is plated onto another agar plate and small discs containing antibiotics are placed on the agar. If the antibiotic disc inhibits the growth of the bacteria then the antibiotic is effective. If the bacteria grow up to the disc then the bacteria are resistant to the actions of the antibiotic. Figure 2.6 shows an agar sensitivity testing plate.

Enzyme-linked immunosorbent assay (ELISA) is used to detect antibody/antigen reactions in the diagnosis of viruses from blood samples. Usually a sample is tested when the patient is in the acute phase of infection, together with a further specimen when the patient is in the convalescent stage. The laboratory

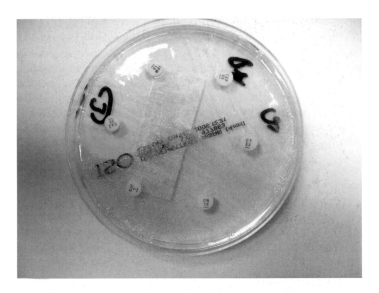

Figure 2.6 Agar sensitivity plate showing antibiotic discs on the plate with resistant micro-organisms growing to touch them.

looks for a four-fold or greater rise in levels of antibody to prove infection.

Immunofluorescence is the staining of micro-organisms with an antibody–dye combination that emits visible light when exposed to ultraviolet light.

ANTIMICROBIAL CHEMOTHERAPY

Antibiotics are substances used to treat infections caused by bacteria. They can either be *bacteriostatic*, in that they do not kill bacteria but prevent them from reproducing, allowing the host defences to kill the micro-organism (e.g. tetracycline); or *bactericidal*, in that they destroy the bacteria (e.g. the aminoglycosides). The first true antibiotic to be successfully used in therapy was penicillin in 1942, in Oxford on a policeman with *Staphylococcus aureus* septicaemia. Unfortunately he died because there were insufficient quantities of the drug for complete treatment. There are now many different groups of antibiotics that act in the following ways:

- **Prevention of cell wall formation** – penicillins, cephalosporins and glycopeptides (e.g. vancomycin, teicoplanin)
- **Alteration of cell membrane permeability** – cyclic peptides (e.g. polymixin)
- **Interference with protein synthesis** – tetracyclines, aminoglycosides, macrolides, fucidic acid and mupirocin
- **Interference with nucleic acid synthesis** – rifamycins and nitrofurans
- **Interference with folic acid synthesis** – sulphonamide, trimethoprim

There are fewer agents available to treat viruses than bacteria. Antiviral agents block the synthesis of RNA or DNA, or they prevent viral uncoating (see Figure 2.4). Acyclovir, given in varicella zoster disease, is an example of an antiviral that blocks DNA synthesis. Other antivirals include those acting against influenza and HIV infection, for example amantadine that acts by preventing uncoating. Antifungal agents include imidazoles, amphotericin B, nystatin and flucytosine. Antiprotozoal agents include quinine and metronidazole.

The choice of antimicrobial treatment is guided by the probable site of infection and the likely causative micro-organism. Where infection is suspected but the causative micro-organism is not yet known then an antibiotic(s) with a broader spectrum of antimicrobial activity is often used. Due to the risk of bacterial resistance developing, as soon as a laboratory result indicating the causative micro-organism is known, an antibiotic with a narrow spectrum of activity should be used (DoH, 2003). To reduce the continuing risk of developing antibiotic resistance, hospitals should have policies on the prescription of antibiotics and these should be strictly adhered to.

BACTERIAL RESISTANCE
Microbial resistance is the ability of a specific micro-organism to withstand a drug that interferes with its growth functions (Cohen and Tartasky, 1997). Bacterial resistance is important in hospital

infection prevention and control as resistance makes infections more difficult and costly to treat. Bacteria are able to resist the actions of antibiotics by:

- Altering the permeability of the cell membrane to prevent the drug from entering the cell
- Preventing the drug from reaching its target site once inside the cell by either pumping out the drug or by trapping the drug inside the bacterial cell
- Inactivating or modifying the drug by use of an enzyme
- Altering the target site for the action of the drug

Bacteria are resistant to antibiotics in a number of ways

Inherent resistance   This is due to the specific bacterial composition in relation to antibiotic action, for example the make-up of the cell wall. It can also be due to the possession of a resistant gene that is only activated when there is exposure to a specific antibiotic.

Genetic mutation   This is spontaneous mutation during the process of multiplication and does not require exposure to antibiotics for this to occur.

Transfer of genetic material   This can occur in one of three ways:

- **Conjugation** (Figure 2.7) A resistant bacteria transfers the resistance gene(s), which may be on a plasmid, to a non-resistant bacteria through a pilus. This is not species specific and the resistance can be passed between different species of micro-organisms.
- **Transformation** (Figure 2.8) A resistant bacteria is killed or dies and its genetic material is released into the environment. A non-resistant bacteria picks up the genetic material from the resistant bacteria, making it resistant.
- **Transduction** (Figure 2.9) A resistant bacteria is infected by a virus (bacteriophage). This bacteriophage acquires the resistant gene from the bacteria during replication. The

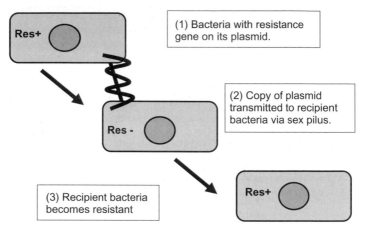

Figure 2.7 Bacterial conjugation.

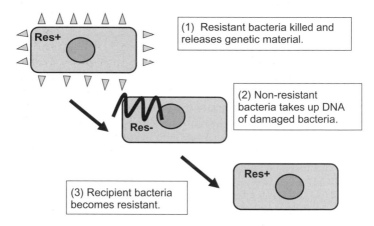

Figure 2.8 Bacterial transformation.

bacteriophage, now carrying the resistant gene, infects a non-resistant bacterial cell. During the process of viral replication, the resistant genetic material is mixed with the bacterial cell's non-resistant DNA. The resistance is then transferred to the

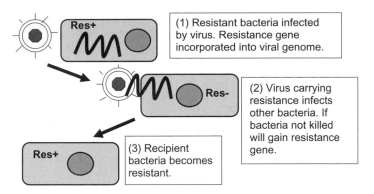

Figure 2.9 Bacterial transduction.

bacterial cell and if it does not die due to viral replication the bacterial cell will then have resistant DNA and will reproduce by binary fission to produce more resistant bacterial cells.

Antibiotic resistance is inevitable. Bacteria have been on the planet for billions of years, having been amongst the earliest of Earth's life forms. To believe that 70 years of antibiotic treatment will reverse the problem of infection is a naive way of thinking. One aim is to slow down the inevitable rise in antimicrobial resistance, wherever possible, and to prevent the transfer of antimicrobial resistant micro-organisms in healthcare situations between patients. Reducing the risk of antibiotic resistance is achieved by:

- Adherence to antibiotic policies
- Prescribing antibiotics with narrow spectrum bacterial activity wherever possible
- Administering antibiotics in accordance with appropriate prescribing with regard to the correct time and dose

ROUTES OF TRANSMISSION

For infections to transmit, there has to be a route for them to move from one human to another. It is important for healthcare staff to understand the routes of micro-organism transmission in hospitals in order to prevent the spread of infection. Micro-organisms are spread in six key ways:

- **Contact** – this can be by either direct or indirect methods. Direct contact is spread from human to human, for example contact with nasopharyngeal secretions or kissing. Indirect contact is spread by either hands, if a healthcare worker handles one patient and then fails to decontaminate their hands before handling another patient, or by contaminated equipment, for example manual handling equipment. This is the most common method by which infections are spread in the hospital environment. Examples of micro-organisms that can be transmitted by this route are *Staphylococcus aureus, Salmonella* spp.

- **Airborne** – this spread can occur by dissemination of small particles (less than 5 micrometres in size) containing micro-organisms. Due to the small particle size, they can remain suspended in the air for some time and can travel on air currents. Examples of micro-organisms that are transmitted by this route are norovirus and influenza. Airborne transmission of aerosols can also occur, for example from contaminated respiratory equipment or air conditioning systems. Dust particles can become airborne during activities that include cleaning and bedmaking. Staphylococci and streptococci are examples of micro-organisms that can be transmitted in airborne dust particles, attached to a 'magic carpet', in this case skin scales of patients and staff. Droplets are another form of airborne transmission. Droplets are generally large (greater than 5 micrometres) particles that are expelled during coughing, sneezing and talking. These are then able to infect susceptible individuals through the mucous membranes of the respiratory tract or the conjunctiva. Due the larger particle size, droplets do not remain suspended in the air for a long period of time and will generally drop to the floor or other horizontal surface within 1–2 metres from the point they were expelled.

- **Faecal-oral** – this is the transmission of enteric infection from the gut of an infected person to the digestive tract of a susceptible individual, for example food poisoning – hepatitis A.

- **Vector** – this is the spread of infection by the means of a living creature, for example malaria or West Nile fever transmission by mosquitoes.

- **Percutaneous** – also referred to as blood to blood transmission, this is the inoculation of an infected body substance into the tissue of a susceptible person. Examples of infections that can be spread by this method include hepatitis B and C or human immunodeficiency syndrome (HIV) transmitted through the sharing of contaminated needles.

- **Vertical** – this is the transmission of infection from mother to baby via the placenta. Varicella zoster is an example of an infection that can be transmitted by this route.

Patients acquiring an infection in hospital will not always acquire this from an outside source; the infection can be from micro-organisms already present on their body. An example of this would be a urinary tract infection due to *Escherichia coli* from a patient's bowel. This is often referred to as self-infection or *endogenous* infection. Where an infection is the result of micro-organisms acquired from an outside source this is referred to as cross infection or *exogenous* infection.

THE INFECTION PROCESS
Micro-organisms are resident at many sites in the human body, for example on the skin or in the vaginal tract. The micro-organisms that normally inhabit these areas are often referred to as commensal organisms or normal flora. If an individual is exposed to other bacteria that then become resident and can multiply at one or more points in the body without causing signs or symptoms of infection, this is often referred to as bacterial colonisation. Truly pathogenic micro-organisms are those that have adapted to overcome the body's defence systems and are able to invade body tissues (Greenwood *et al.*, 2002). Infection is characterised by reactions in the body including pyrexia and tachycardia.

For micro-organisms to initiate an infection, they must gain entry to the body. This can be achieved in several ways:

- Through a break in, or damage to, the integrity of the skin, for example a surgical incision (staphylococci), accidental injury (streptococci, tetanus), intravenous cannulae (staphylococci), bites (streptococci, rabies), or burns (pseudomonas)
- Through inhalation of aerosols or droplets (pneumococci – the primary cause of pneumonia, influenza, chickenpox)
- Through ingestion of contaminated food or water (salmonella, campylobacter, hepatitis A, norovirus)
- Through sexual contact (hepatitis B and C, chlamydia)
- Through the urinary tract (*Escherichia coli*, other Gram negative bacteria)
- Through inoculation into the bloodstream or by contaminated blood products (hepatitis B and C)
- Meningitis usually occurs following colonisation or infection of the upper respiratory tract, progressing to infection of the blood and penetration of the cerebrospinal fluid, for example *Neisseria meningitidis*.

THE IMMUNE RESPONSE

The human body is protected from infection by an immune system that has non-specific response, which includes a number of mechanisms that provide general protection against infection and specific responses that provide protection against specific micro-organisms.

Non-specific immune actions to prevent invasion by micro-organisms

The first line of immune response is protection against invasion from micro-organisms. This is achieved by:

- **The skin** – this provides a tough, waterproof barrier when intact. The skin is colonised by its own resident micro-organisms, for example *Staphylococcus epidermidis*, which protects against colonisation by harmful bacteria. The secretions from the sweat and sebaceous glands contain antibacterial properties.

- **Mucous membranes** – the mucous membranes lining the mouth, urethra, gastro-intestinal tract, female genital tract and the respiratory tract produce secretions that entrap micro-organisms until other functions of the immune system can address them (Keyworth, 2000). The cilia of the respiratory tract move mucous and entrapped micro-organisms away from the lower respiratory tract towards the mouth.

- **Secretions and excretions** – some of the body secretions, for example tears and nasal mucus, contain lysozyme. This has antibacterial properties. Vaginal secretions and gastric secretions are acidic, making the environment non-conducive to bacterial multiplication. The flushing action of urine during voiding from the bladder helps to remove micro-organisms that may be colonising the urinary tract.

Non-specific immune response following microbial invasion

If micro-organisms successfully breach the body's first lines of defence, the immune system then employs other functions:

- **Inflammatory response** – the body's inflammatory response mechanisms respond to the presence of a foreign body in tissues, including micro-organisms. The classical signs and symptoms of inflammations are swelling, tenderness, redness, pain and heat. The process of inflammation begins with dilation of the capillaries that then allows white and red blood cells to leak out from the blood vessels into the tissue. Fibrin is also released from the capillaries, which then forms a mesh aimed at preventing micro-organisms from spreading further into the tissues.

- **Phagocytosis** – two of the body's white blood cells, neutrophils and mononuclear phagocytes, are also released from the blood vessels in the vicinity of the invading micro-organisms. Their role is to engulf foreign bodies and to ingest them by the action of enzymes.

- **Interferons** – in response to viral infections, interferons are produced by cells, which act on other cells in the vicinity of the virus infected cell to make them more resistant to the actions of the virus.

- **The complement system** – this enhances phagocytosis (a process known as opsonisation), increases the permeability of blood vessels, attracts phagocytes to the site of micro-organism invasion and damages the cell walls of invading foreign bodies. The complement system is a series of proteins and enzymes that are inactive in the blood until activated by the presence of a foreign body.

- **Fever** – a rise in temperature may increase the body's ability to repair itself and enhance the immune response (Wilson, 1995). An increase in temperature may also serve to help the body destroy micro-organisms that are pathogenic to man, which often have an optimum breeding temperature of 37°C.

The specific immune response
In addition to the processes of the non-specific immune response, lymphocytes, produced by the bone marrow, have specific action against invading micro-organisms. B-lymphocytes are involved in humoral immunity and are active in bacterial infections. T-lymphocytes are involved in cell-mediated immunity and are active in viral infections and tuberculosis.

- **Humoral immunity** – B-lymphocytes originate from the stem cells in bone marrow and are responsible for the production of antibodies. Antibodies are Y-shaped proteins, also called immunoglobulins, that have several functions. B-lymphocytes have different antibodies on their surfaces that are designed to attach to different antigens (the molecules of the cell wall of invading micro-organism). The stem of the Y in an immunoglobulin activates the complement system and assists phagocytes to attach to and engulf invading micro-organisms. The head of the Y binds to the specific antigen and then produces numerous clones of itself, which can then develop into plasma cells. These plasma cells manufacture and release antibodies but die after a short time. Some develop into memory cells, which remain in the bloodstream for many years and are then ready to act rapidly in response to infection by the same antigen in the future. There are five classes of immunoglobulin, which are produced at different times in the

Table 2.4 Actions of immunoglobulins.

Immunoglobulin	Action and activity
Immunoglobulin A	Blocks the adherence of bacteria and viruses to mucous membranes. Secreted in the gut, respiratory tract, tears and saliva.
Immunoglobulin D	Present on the surface of some circulating B-cells. Accounts for less than 1% of circulating antibody. More prolific in childhood but action is relatively unknown.
Immunoglobulin E	Can be found attached to mast cells and basophils. Triggers the release of histamine.
Immunoglobulin G	Assists in opsonisation and activation of complement. Accounts for approximately 75% of circulating antibody. Can cross the placenta in the late stages of pregnancy. Appears one to two weeks after infection and may be produced for up to a year after infection.
Immunoglobulin M	Assists in complement activation and phagocytosis. The first immunoglobulin to appear after infection.

immune process and have different activities and actions (Table 2.4).

- **Cell-mediated immunity** – T-lymphocytes also originate from the bone marrow but are developed in the thymus gland. They protect the body from intracellular bacterial infections, viral infections, some fungal infections and parasites. T-lymphocytes release lymphokines, which activate macrophages in the local tissue. Together the T-lymphocytes and the activated macrophages also act by recognising cells that have become foreign due to virus infection. T-lymphocytes, when activated, differentiate into different types of T-cells:

  — T-helper cells (also known as CD4), which assist in the production of antibodies by B-lymphocytes
  — T-suppressor cells (also known as CD8), which balance the activity of the helper cells to prevent cell damage and excessive reaction
  — Natural killer cells, which destroy foreign and infected cells

— Memory T-cells, which remain for many years and are ready to mount an instant response if exposed to the same antigen in the future

Vaccination and immunisation

Natural immunity occurs with prior exposure to a micro-organism, through the processes described previously in this chapter. It is possible for individuals to be immune to infections, for example chickenpox, without being aware that they have previously been infected if the primary infection has been sub-clinical.

Passive acquired immunity occurs when an individual is provided with antibodies from another source. This could be via the placenta in passing immunity from mother to child, or by the administration of antibodies harvested from the blood of other immune individuals.

Active acquired immunity occurs when an individual is exposed to either a small dose or an inactivated dose of an antigen. This is the process that is used in vaccinations.

SCENARIO

The microbiology laboratory scientist contacts you with an urgent blood culture result for a patient who had undergone surgery and has signs of a wound infection as well as general sepsis. The laboratory scientist advises you that the blood culture shows Gram positive cocci but that at present they have not identified the specific bacteria. What is this bacteria most likely to be?

Staphylococcus aureus is a common cause of hospital-acquired wound infection. *S. aureus* is a Gram positive coccus. As the patient has signs and symptoms of a wound infection this would be one of the most likely causes; *Streptococcus pyogenes* could also be a cause of this infection. The patient would be started on antibiotic treatment that would be effective against Gram positive cocci at this stage. When final identification and antibiotic sensitivities of the bacteria were known, the antibiotics would be reviewed as to their appropriateness and effectiveness.

SUMMARY

Either bacteria, viruses, fungi or protozoa can cause human infections. Spread of micro-organisms in hospitals can be by a number of routes, including airborne, contact, faecal-oral or percutaneous. Micro-organisms do not always cause infection in humans; some bacteria are always present on the human body, some may be acquired but only lead to colonisation not infection. Micro-organisms can be treated with antimicrobials but some have inbuilt or acquired resistance to commonly used treatments. Humans have an immune system, which operates at a number of levels, to protect from specific infections and micro-organisms in general.

REFERENCES

Cohen, F.L. and Tartasky, D. (1997) Microbial resistance to drug therapy: a review. *American Journal of Infection Control*, **25** (1), 51–64.

Department of Health (2003) *Winning Ways: Working Together to Reduce Healthcare Associated Infection in England*. Department of Health, London.

Greenwood, D., Slack, R.C.B. and Peutherer, J.F. (2002) *Medical Microbiology: a Guide to Microbial Infections, Pathogenesis, Immunity, Laboratory Diagnosis and Control*. Churchill Livingstone, London.

Keyworth, N. (2000) Introduction to the immune system. In: *Infection Control: Science, Management and Practice* (ed. J. McCulloch). Whurr Publishers, London.

Wilson, J. (1995) *Infection Control in Clinical Practice*. Baillière Tindall, London.

FURTHER READING

Manojilovic, G. (2003) Immunosuppressive diseases. In: *Infection Control in the Community* (eds J. Lawrence and D. May). Churchill Livingstone, Edinburgh.

3 | Specimen Collection

INTRODUCTION

The interpretive nature of microbiology means that it is vitally important for specimens sent to the laboratory to be collected, stored and transported correctly. This chapter covers practical aspects of common specimens sent for laboratory analysis.

LEARNING OBJECTIVES

By the end of this chapter you will be able to:

❑ Identify key safety and quality principles for collection, storage and transport of specimens
❑ Describe practices related to collection of microbiological specimens including:

— Wound swabs
— Faecal specimens
— Urine specimens
— Nasopharyngeal aspirate
— Blood cultures

SPECIMEN COLLECTION, STORAGE AND TRANSPORT PRINCIPLES

Specimens should only be obtained and sent for processing if there is a clinical need for the investigation to be carried out. Patient consent should always be obtained before taking specimens and for certain laboratory tests (e.g. testing for human immunodeficiency virus) counselling of the patient is a vital precursor to ensure that the implications of a positive test have been considered. The accuracy of a test result can be dependent on the quality of the specimen obtained as well as the time taken for transportation and the method by which it is stored and transported.

Safety of staff obtaining specimens and laboratory staff who will be processing the specimen should be considered, as specimens for microbiological examination are not only hazardous in themselves, but may also contain micro-organisms that have specific handling requirements under Control of Substances Hazardous to Health Regulations (HSE, 1999). When processing and reporting on microbiological specimens it is important that sufficient clinical information is provided for the laboratory as micro-organisms may be part of the normal body bacteria at certain sites but at other sites may have the potential to cause infection. The following principles should be applied to collection, storage and handling of specimens for microbiological examination:

- Patient consent should be obtained before collecting the specimen.
- Specimens should be sent on clinical need only.
- Staff collecting specimens should wear protective clothing in accordance with standard precautions (see Chapter 5).
- Specimen containers should be stored in a manner that reduces the risk of their contamination.
- Specimens should be safely contained in a leak-proof container.
- The container lid should be checked to ensure it is fitted correctly.
- The patient's details should be correctly and fully completed on the specimen container.
- The specimen container should be enclosed in an outer container (often a plastic bag).
- The specimen request form should be fully completed to include:

  — Patient's name, ward and/or department
  — Hospital number and/or date of birth
  — Date and time of specimen collection
  — Specimen type in sufficient detail (for example, 'mid-stream urine' as opposed to just stating 'urine')
  — Diagnosis and/or signs and symptoms

- Relevant history (for example recent foreign travel)
- Current and recent antimicrobial treatment
- Contact details for requesting practitioner and for practitioner or medical staff in charge of the patient's care
- Whether the patient has a known biohazard condition (for example tuberculosis, as processing of the specimen may need to be undertaken in a controlled environment)

- The specimen request form should not be placed immediately adjacent to the primary specimen container, to prevent contamination of the form in the event of leakage.
- The outside container should be kept free from contamination.
- Specimens should be transported to the laboratory at the earliest opportunity.
- Specimens that require refrigeration whilst awaiting collection should be placed in a designated specimen fridge and not in a food or drug refrigerator.
- Specimens should be transported to the laboratory via a designated collection service wherever possible.
- If nursing or other staff are transporting specimens to the laboratory they must not be carried in pockets due to risk of spillage. A designated specimen container that is leak proof and carries the United Nations symbol for hazardous substances, together with contact details in event of loss, should be used.
- Specimens must not be sent to the laboratory through internal mail systems.
- Specimens being sent externally by Royal Mail must be sent in Post Office approved packaging.
- The collection and sending of a specimen should be noted in the patient's clinical record (WHO, 2000; HSE, 2003; Dougherty and Lister, 2004).

WOUND SPECIMENS

Wound swabs may be taken to confirm the presence of potentially pathogenic micro-organisms if a wound appears to be clinically infected, in order to determine appropriate antibiotic therapy. Swabs should only be sent if clinically relevant, as laboratories may not process specimens if the patient is not unwell. Swabs may be taken to detect colonisation with clinically relevant micro-organisms, for example meticillin resistant *Staphylococcus aureus*, but in general should not be taken to detect colonisation alone.

Clinical signs of infection that may indicate the need for taking a wound swab include:

- Change in pain of the wound and/or surrounding area (NB patients with diabetes may have reduced pain sensation)
- Elevated blood glucose in persons with diabetes
- Delayed healing/prolonged length of healing in relation to the type of wound
- Hot, red and inflamed wound +/− surrounding area (cellulitic)
- Increasing volume of exudate or change in appearance of exudates
- Deteriorating wound condition, for example increased size of wound or amount of necrotic tissue
- Pyrexia
- Malodour/offensive smelling

When collecting swabs from a surface wound avoid areas where there are signs of healing. If a swab is to be taken from a sinus tract the specimen should be taken from as close to the base of the sinus tract as possible. If the specimen is from an abscess, pus obtained using a syringe and needle may be the most appropriate sampling method; local laboratory guidelines should be consulted.

Procedure for obtaining a wound swab

- Inform patient of the need to take the swab and obtain permission.
- Prepare equipment as required.
- Decontaminate hands with soap and water.
- Using an aseptic technique, remove any dressings and clean away any excess dressing materials (e.g. hydrocolloids, hydrogels) or faecal soiling present. In the absence of any dressing material or soiling the wound should not be cleaned before taking the swab.

- Moisten the wound swab with 0.9% sterile saline if the area to be swabbed is dry.
- The specimen should be taken by gently rotating the swab on the infected area of the wound.
- Care should be taken to not contaminate other areas of the wound.
- Return the swab to the container with transport medium, taking care not to contaminate the swab or the outside of the container.
- Continue with appropriate wound care and complete the dressing procedure.
- Remove protective clothing and decontaminate hands.
- Complete patient's details clearly on the swab container with patient's name, date of birth, hospital number, source of swab, date and time the sample was taken.
- Complete the laboratory form correctly.
- Check that the details on the specimen container and the form are identical.
- Place the swab in a plastic specimen bag with the form either attached to the outside or in a separate pocket.
- Place the swab in the designated collection area.
- Decontaminate hands.
- Document procedure in patient records (Donovan, 1998; Gilchrist, 2000; Kingsley, 2003; Dougherty and Lister, 2004; Health Protection Agency, 2006).

URINE SPECIMENS

Urine specimens are taken in patients who have symptomatic urinary tract infection to guide antibiotic therapy. Occasionally urine specimens are taken as part of a screening process for clinically relevant micro-organisms prior to surgery, for example surgery on the urinary tract or for prosthetic implants. Urine specimens should not be taken as routine in patients with catheters unless there are signs of infection.

The following signs and symptoms may indicate a urinary tract infection and the need for obtaining a urine specimen:

- Urgency
- Frequency

- Dysuria
- Loin pain
- Loin or suprapubic tenderness
- Pyrexia greater than 38°C
- Haematuria
- Pyuria

Procedure for obtaining a mid-stream or clean-catch urine specimen

- Wherever possible a mid-stream urine should be obtained in preference to a clean-catch specimen.
- Inform the patient of the need to take the urine specimen and obtain consent.
- The urethral area, including the perineal area for women, should be thoroughly cleaned with soap and water to minimise the risk of contamination.
- If assisting the patient, decontaminate hands and wear non-sterile gloves.
- Ask the patient to commence micturition into the toilet, commode or bedpan then insert a sterile bowl or clinically clean disposable multi-cup into the stream of urine before the flow stops.
- For clean-catch specimens insert the sterile bowl or clinically clean multi-cup into the commode, toilet or bedpan and ask the patient to micturate into the bowl.
- Ensure patients are offered hand washing opportunities on completion of micturition.
- Transfer the sample into a sterile universal specimen container and secure the lid for safe transport. Five to ten ml of urine is generally sufficient for microbiological examination.
- Remove protective clothing and decontaminate hands.
- Complete patient's details clearly on the specimen container with patient's name, date of birth, hospital number, specimen type, date and time the sample taken.
- Complete the laboratory request form accurately; check that the information on the form and the specimen container tally.
- Document clearly on the specimen form whether the sample is mid-stream or clean-catch.

- Place the specimen in a plastic specimen bag with the form either attached to the outside or in a separate pocket.
- Place the specimen in the designated collection area.
- Decontaminate hands.
- Document procedure in patient records. (World Health Organization, 2000; Dougherty and Lister, 2004)

Procedure for obtaining a urine specimen from a child or infant wearing nappies

- Inform child and parents of the process of the investigation and obtain consent for the procedure.
- Decontaminate hands with soap and water.
- Thoroughly cleanse the urethral area, including perineum area for females, with soap and water to minimise the degree of contamination.
- Place a sterile cotton wool ball or urine collecting pad into the nappy where the child would micturate or attach a uri-bag and secure the nappy.
- Once the child has passed urine, remove the nappy.
- Wearing *sterile gloves*, squeeze urine into suitable specimen container and secure the lid for safe transport to the laboratories. Five to ten ml should be sufficient for microbiological investigation.
- If collecting the urine sample from a uri-bag, decant the specimen into a specimen container.
- Decontaminate hands with soap and water.
- Complete patient's details clearly on the specimen container with the patient's name, date of birth, hospital number, specimen type, date and time the sample was taken.
- Complete the laboratory request form accurately; check that the information on the form and the specimen container tally.
- Document clearly on the specimen form whether the sample is clean-catch or from sterile cotton pad.
- Place the specimen in a plastic specimen bag with the form either attached to the outside or in a separate pocket.
- Place the specimen in the designated collection area.
- Decontaminate hands.

• Document procedure in patient records. (Ahmad *et al.*, 1991; Feasey, 1999; Farrell *et al.*, 2002)

Procedure for obtaining a catheter specimen of urine

• If there is no urine in the tubing, clamp the tubing until enough urine has collected for testing.
• Decontaminate hands.
• Don non-sterile gloves.
• Clean rubber access port with alcohol swab to reduce the risk of introducing contamination.
• Using a sterile 10 ml syringe (and needle if the catheter does not have a needle-free port), aspirate the required amount of urine from rubber port.
• Five to ten ml should be sufficient for microbiological investigation.
• Do not take specimens from the emptying port of catheter bag as this can provide a false result.
• Re-clean the access port with alcohol swab to reduce contamination of the access point and cross infection.
• Place the urine specimen in a sterile universal container.
• Ensure the lid is secured firmly to prevent leakage.
• Unclamp the catheter tubing to allow urine drainage to continue.
• Discard the syringe and needle, if used, into a sharps bin.
• Remove gloves and decontaminate hands.
• Label specimen container with patient's name, hospital number, ward, date/time of collection and specimen type.
• Complete the laboratory request form accurately; check that the information on the form and the specimen container tally.
• Document clearly on the specimen form that this is a catheter specimen of urine.
• Place the specimen in a plastic specimen bag with the form either attached to the outside or in a separate pocket.
• Place the specimen in the designated collection area.
• Decontaminate hands.
• Document procedure in patient records. (World Health Organization, 2000; Dougherty and Lister, 2004)

FAECAL SPECIMENS

Faecal specimens for microbiological analysis are taken to identify bacterial, viral and parasitic causes of gastro-intestinal infection. Faecal specimens may also be taken for other laboratory analysis purposes, for example testing for occult blood; the method for sample collection and handling in these circumstances is the same as for sample collection for microbiological analysis. Microbiological examination of faeces is generally undertaken when patients are experiencing diarrhoea, that is frequent episodes of loose watery stools. Microbiological examination is also undertaken during outbreak investigations and to confirm clearance of specific enteric infections, for example, *Escherichia coli* 0157. Segments of tapeworm can be easily identified in faeces and should be sent to pathology for identification. Include the head of the tapeworm, if present, as this will aid laboratory identification. Patients suspected of having amoebic dysentery should have a stool specimen sent to the laboratory *as soon as possible*, as the parasite that causes amoebic dysentery is difficult to identify once dead.

Procedure for obtaining a faecal specimen

- Inform patient of the need to take the specimen, explain the procedure and obtain permission.
- Ask the patient to defecate into a clean bedpan, commode, or, if a child, a potty or nappy.
- Wearing gloves and aprons, use the scoop inside the faecal collection pot to place enough faecal matter to fill one third of the pot, or the size of a walnut, into the pot.
- Dispose of faecal matter in bedpan, commode, potty or nappy and disinfect any reusable equipment.
- Remove and dispose of gloves.
- Decontaminate hands with soap and water if patient has diarrhoea.
- Complete patient's details clearly on the specimen container with patient's name, date of birth, hospital number, source of swab, date and time the sample was taken.
- Complete the laboratory form correctly.

- If the sample is being examined for possible *Clostridium difficile* infection it is important that the antibiotic history is clearly stated. If the sample is being sent because viral gastroenteritis is suspected this should be clearly stated on the laboratory form. If the patient has had recent foreign travel this should also be noted.
- Check that the details on the specimen container and the form are identical.
- Place the specimen in a plastic specimen bag with the form either attached to the outside or in a separate pocket.
- Place the specimen in the designated collection area.
- Decontaminate hands.
- Document procedure in patient records. (World Health Organization, 2000)

BLOOD CULTURES

Blood cultures are taken to identify micro-organisms causing bloodstream infection, which may include bacteria and fungi. The presence of micro-organisms in blood is referred to as bacteraemia; where these micro-organisms are causing symptoms of bloodstream infection this is referred to as septicaemia. Blood cultures should be taken if a patient is suspected of having bacteraemia displaying signs and symptoms including fever, chills, rigors and hypotension. Wherever possible blood cultures should be taken before antimicrobial therapy is given as this may impede microbial growth and lead to a false negative sample. It is important that an aseptic technique is followed when obtaining blood cultures as contamination of the specimen can lead to a false positive result. Blood cultures should not be drawn from an existing intravenous access device unless this is being obtained as part of the process to diagnose catheter related bloodstream infection.

Procedure for obtaining a blood culture from a peripheral vein

- Inform patient of the need to take the blood sample and where possible obtain consent from the patient.

- Collect required equipment including gloves, blood culture bottles, two antiseptic wipes, for skin cleansing and for disinfecting the injection caps of the bottles, sharps container for disposal of sharps, tourniquet.
- Decontaminate hands and apply tourniquet.
- Apply gloves.
- Cleanse skin at venepuncture site with antiseptic wipe and allow to dry before proceeding.
- Disinfect injection cap of blood culture bottles with an antiseptic wipe and allow to dry.
- Obtain blood sample using recommended hospital method; a vacuum collection system, for example Vacutainer, should be used in preference to the use of a needle and syringe, followed by injection through the culture bottle caps to reduce risk of needlestick injury and contamination of the specimen.
- If a syringe and needle are used, the needle should be changed before injecting the blood through the culture bottle caps if a safety needle is used.
- Dispose of sharps used into sharps container at the point of use.
- Remove gloves, dispose of waste in appropriate container.
- Decontaminate hands.
- Complete patient's details clearly on the blood culture bottles with the patient's name, date of birth, hospital number, specimen type, date and time the sample was taken.
- Complete the laboratory request form accurately; check that the information on the form and the specimen container tally.
- Place the specimen in a plastic specimen bag with the form either attached to the outside or in a separate pocket.
- Arrange immediate transport to the laboratory or incubate in a designated specimen incubator locally.
- Decontaminate hands.
- Document procedure in patient records. (Hall and Lyman, 2006)

Obtaining blood cultures through an intravascular line
Wherever possible, indwelling intravascular lines alone should not be used to obtain blood cultures as colonisation of the

intravascular line could lead to false positive results (Baer, 2003). If it is necessary to use an existing line the following procedure and an aseptic technique (see Chapter 8) should be followed:

- Inform patient of the need to take the blood sample and where possible obtain consent from the patient.
- Collect required equipment including gloves, blood culture bottles, two sterile syringes, two antiseptic swabs, for cleansing the hub and for disinfecting the injection caps of the bottles, sharps container for disposal of sharps.
- Disinfect injection cap of blood culture bottles with an antiseptic wipe and allow to dry.
- Decontaminate hands.
- Apply gloves.
- Cleanse the access port of the intravascular line with an antiseptic wipe for at least five seconds (cleansing time may be longer if a needleless valve is in place – refer to manufacturers' guidance).
- Attach a sterile syringe to cleansed port and withdraw 5–10 ml of blood; place to one side to discard.
- Attach a second sterile syringe to cleansed port and withdraw required amount of blood.
- Recap line port if not using a needleless valve.
- Transfer blood sample to culture bottles, taking care not to contaminate the sample and avoiding needlestick injury.
- Dispose of sharps used into sharps container at the point of use.
- Remove gloves, dispose of waste in appropriate container.
- Decontaminate hands.
- Complete patient's details clearly on the blood culture bottles with the patient's name, date of birth, hospital number, specimen type, date and time the sample was taken.
- Complete the laboratory request form accurately; check that the information on the form and the specimen container tally.
- Place the specimen in a plastic specimen bag with the form either attached to the outside or in a separate pocket.
- Arrange immediate transport to the laboratory or incubate in a designated specimen incubator locally.

- Decontaminate hands.
- Document procedure in patient records.

NASOPHARYNGEAL ASPIRATES

Nasopharyngeal specimens are mainly taken to detect viruses causing respiratory tract infection, including respiratory syncytial virus and influenza. The quantity of virus will be greater whilst patients are symptomatic of infection with production of mucus and, therefore, detection of virus is more likely. Specimens from asymptomatic patients are likely to be of limited clinical benefit and due to the unpleasantness of this investigation should only be obtained if there is specific need, for example in determining cessation of isolation precautions in an oncology setting. Nasopharyngeal specimens may be obtained by a nasal wash using a syringe and sterile saline (Dougherty and Lister, 2004). However, they are more likely to be obtained by the suction assisted nasal aspiration method.

Procedure for suction assisted nasal aspiration

- Inform patient of the need to take the sample, explain procedure and obtain consent.
- Collect required equipment including gloves, suction pump, sterile suction catheter, mucus trap and viral transport medium if required.
- Decontaminate hands and assemble equipment.
- Apply gloves.
- Turn on suction but do not apply suction whilst inserting the catheter.
- Insert the suction catheter via the nose to the pharynx (Figure 3.1).
- Apply the suction and using a rotating motion slowly withdraw the suction catheter.
- If rinsing with viral transport medium is required, continue to apply the suction and aspirate 10–20 ml of transport medium into the mucus trap.
- Taking care not to contaminate equipment or the outside of the mucus trap with secretions, turn off suction and connect the tubing to the open end of the mucus trap to seal the specimen in, preventing leakage.

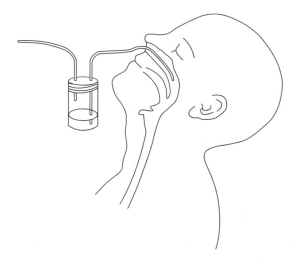

Figure 3.1 Suction assisted nasopharyngeal aspiration (reproduced with kind permission from Dougherty and Lister, 2004).

- Remove gloves, dispose of waste in appropriate container.
- Decontaminate hands.
- Complete patient's details clearly on the mucus trap and include specimen type, date and time the sample was taken.
- Complete the laboratory request form accurately; check that the information on the form and the specimen container tally.
- Place the specimen in a plastic specimen bag with the form either attached to the outside or in a separate pocket.
- Place the specimen in the designated specimen collection area.
- Decontaminate hands.
- Document procedure in patient records.

METICILLIN RESISTANT *STAPHYLOCOCCUS AUREUS* (MRSA) SCREENING SPECIMENS

Specimens are taken to detect carriage of MRSA either before a patient is admitted to hospital or undergoes specific treatments, as part of a screening process in event of cases or an outbreak of MRSA and to check for clearance of MRSA skin carriage. Sampling the nose is an essential part of an MRSA screening protocol, as most patients who are colonised at other sites will have MRSA in the nose (DoH, 2006). In addition to nasal swabs, samples are often taken from the following sites:

- Throat
- Perineum
- Hairline
- Axillae
- Groin
- Wounds or broken skin
- Urine specimens if catheterised

When taking samples from the nose, throat and intact skin the swab can be moistened in sterile 0.9% saline solution before sampling as this assists in the transfer of bacteria from the sampling site to the swab. When sampling the nose, the moistened swab should be rotated in the anterior nares of both nostrils.

THROAT SWABS

Throat swabs may be taken to detect the presence of either bacteria or viruses. Viral swabs should not be placed into bacterial swab transport medium; instead they should be transported in a dry sterile transport container to the laboratory.

Procedure for obtaining a throat swab

- Inform patient of the need to take the swab, explain the procedure and obtain permission.
- Prepare equipment as required.
- Decontaminate hands with soap and water.
- Position the patient facing a strong light source and depress the tongue with a disposable spatula to ensure good vision of the area to be swabbed.
- If there is obvious exudate or a lesion, gently sample the area; if none is obvious, gently swab the tonsillar fossa (Figure 3.2).

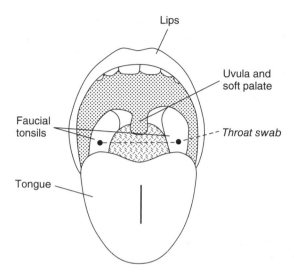

Figure 3.2 Sampling area for a throat swab (reproduced with kind permission from Dougherty and Lister, 2004).

- Care should be taken not to contaminate the swab by contact with the tongue of the oral mucosa on removal.
- Return the swab to the container with transport medium if a bacteriology sample, or the plain transport container if a viral sample, taking care not to contaminate the swab or the outside of the container.
- Decontaminate hands.
- Complete patient's details clearly on the swab container with patient's name, date of birth, hospital number, source of swab, date and time the sample was taken.
- Complete the laboratory form correctly.
- Check that the details on the specimen container and the form are identical.
- Place the swab in a plastic specimen bag with the form either attached to the outside or in a separate pocket.
- Place the swab in the designated collection area.
- Decontaminate hands.

- Document procedure in patient records. (World Health Organization, 2000; Dougherty and Lister, 2004)

SPUTUM

Sputum specimens are sent for microbiological analysis to detect bacteria and viruses. Sputum specimens may also be sent for other purposes, such as histological investigation, in which case the method of collection and transport is the same as for microbiological analysis. For certain investigations, for example tuberculosis, it may be necessary to send more than one consecutive sample. Sputum should be sent for microbiological culture if the patient has signs or symptoms of a lower respiratory tract infection including:

- Productive cough
- Blood stained sputum
- Pyrexia greater than 38°C

When obtaining sputum samples for tuberculosis, staff may need to wear a mask or respirator in line with hospital policy. Collection of sputum samples by induction should never be carried out in an open ward environment where immunocompromised patients are present; it must always be undertaken in a single room, preferably with negative pressure ventilation (the Interdepartmental Working Group on Tuberculosis, 1998).

Procedure for obtaining a sputum sample

- Inform patient of the need to take the sample, explain the procedure and obtain permission.
- Prepare equipment as required, including mask or respirator if appropriate.
- Provide patient with sterile universal container and explain to patient the need to expectorate sputum into the pot.
- Wearing appropriate protective clothing, once patient has expectorated, visually examine sample to ensure it contains sputum and not saliva.
- Ensure lid is securely fastened on universal container to prevent leakage.

- Remove protective clothing and decontaminate hands.
- Complete patient's details clearly on the specimen container with patient's name, date of birth, hospital number, source of specimen, date and time the sample was taken.
- Complete the laboratory form correctly.
- If the sample is for known or suspected tuberculosis, the bio-hazard notification on the form and specimen container must be used.
- Check that the details on the specimen container and the form are identical.
- Place the specimen in a plastic specimen bag with the form either attached to the outside or in a separate pocket.
- Place the specimen in the designated collection area.
- Decontaminate hands.
- Document procedure in patient records. (World Health Organization, 2000)

SCENARIO

Mrs Wells is a 44-year-old lady who has undergone an abdominal hysterectomy. She has had a urinary catheter in situ but this has now been removed. What would be the indications to send a urine specimen?

Bacteria could be present in Mrs Wells' urine without her actually having a urinary tract infection. A urine specimen should only be sent if Mrs Wells showed signs or symptoms of an infection, which may include loin pain, dysuria, frequency, urgency and pyrexia.

SUMMARY

Specimens for microbiological investigation should only be taken when there is evidence of infection or clinical need. Safe collection and transport is important to prevent infection of other patients, nurses, porters and laboratory staff. Following guidelines on specimen collection is vital to ensure the microbiology laboratory are able to accurately identify micro-organisms and to reduce the risk of false positive samples.

REFERENCES

Ahmad, T., Vickers, D., Campbell, S. *et al.* (1991) Urine collection from disposable nappies. *Lancet*, **338**, 674–676.

Baer, D.M. (2003) Answering your questions: blood cultures collected from IV line. *Medical Laboratory Observer*, January.

Department of Health (2006) *Screening for Meticillin Resistant Staphylococcus aureus (MRSA) Colonisation: a Strategy for NHS Trusts: a Summary of Best Practice*. Available at: www.dh.gov.uk/reducingmrsa (accessed 22 November 2006).

Donovan, S. (1998) Wound infection and wound swabbing. *Professional Nurse*, **13** (August, 11), 157–159.

Dougherty, L. and Lister, S. (eds) (2004) *The Royal Marsden Hospital Manual of Clinical Nursing Procedures* (sixth edition). Blackwell Publishing, Oxford.

Farrell, M., Devine, K., Lancaster, G. *et al.* (2002) A method comparison study to assess the reliability of urine collection pads as a means of obtaining urine specimens from non-toilet trained children for microbiological investigation. *Journal of Advanced Nursing*, **37**, 387–393.

Feasey, S. (1999) Are Newcastle urine collection pads suitable as a means of collecting urine specimens from infants? *Pediatric Nurse*, **11**, 17–21.

Gilchrist, B. (2000) Taking a wound swab. *Nursing Times Plus*, **96** (4), 2.

Hall, K.K. and Lyman, J.A. (2006) Updated review of blood culture contamination. *Clinical Microbiology Reviews*, **19**, 788–802.

Health and Safety Executive (1999) *Control of Substances Hazardous to Health (COSHH) (Amendments) Act*. Health and Safety Executive, London.

Health and Safety Executive (2003) *Safe Working and the Prevention of Infection in Clinical Laboratories and Similar Facilities*. HSE Books, London.

Health Protection Agency (2006) Venous leg ulcers: infection diagnosis and microbiological investigation. Available at: http://www.hpa.org.uk/infections/topics_az/primary_care_guidance/leg_ulcer_guide_070906.pdf (accessed 23 November 2006).

Kingsley, A. (2003) Audit of wound swab sampling: why protocols could improve practice. *Professional Nurse*, **18** (6), 338–343.

The Interdepartmental Working Group on Tuberculosis (1998) *UK Guidance on Prevention and Control of (1) HIV-related Tuberculosis (2) Drug-resistant, including Multiple Drug Resistant Tuberculosis*. Department of Health, London.

World Health Organization (2000) Guidelines for collection of clinical specimens during field investigations of outbreaks. Available at: http://www.who.int/csr/resources/publications/surveillance/whocdscsredc2004.pdf (accessed 23 November 2006).

Risk Assessment

4

INTRODUCTION

To determine appropriate infection control practices, the first step involves an assessment of the risk of transmission of infection. Patients in hospital can be both at risk of acquiring an infection as well as being a risk for transmission of infection to other patients. Risk assessment is the first step in devising plans of management and care. This chapter covers the assessment of risk individual patients have of acquiring an infection, as well as the risk of transmitting infection.

LEARNING OBJECTIVES

By the end of this chapter you will be able to:

❏ Identify key factors that increase a patient's risk of infection
❏ Assess the risk of infection transmission from an infected patient
❏ Devise a plan of care for patients at risk of infection
❏ Devise a plan of management to prevent infection transmission from an infected patient.

Risk management is an important process in healthcare to reduce the risk of adverse incidents, including infection (Pratt *et al.*, 2002). Assessment of infection risk can be carried out in relation to most healthcare activities, from both the perspective of the healthcare worker and the patient. Proactive risk assessment processes can be used to assess the risk of infection to individual patients and to plan their care accordingly, or can be used to assess the risk of transmission from an infected patient to other patients.

ASSESSING INFECTION RISK TO INDIVIDUAL PATIENTS

Factors that increase risk of infection can be categorised according to whether they are general factors, local factors, invasive procedures, drugs or disease related (Bowell, 1992).

General factors

General factors on an individual basis may not significantly increase risk of infection, but may have an effect in combination.

- **Age** – babies and young children will be at increased risk of infection due to the immaturity of their immune system, whereas for elderly patients the efficacy of their immune system can be reduced. Increasing age is a risk factor for urinary tract infection (Wilkie *et al.*, 1992).

- **Nutrition** – a poor diet can increase the risk of infection, as essential nutrients to support tissue healing and repair may be lacking. Weight loss within the preceding six months can increase risk of surgical site infection (Malone *et al.*, 2002).

- **Mobility** – the patient with limited mobility or who is immobile will be at greater risk of lower respiratory infection (Tablan *et al.*, 2003).

- **Hygiene** – the patient who needs assistance with general hygiene is likely to have greater contact with healthcare workers during their hospital stay and could therefore be at greater risk from contact transmission of infection. Patients who are incontinent of faeces and/or urine could be at increased risk of endogenous infection, for example urinary tract infection due to *Escherichia coli* present in their own faeces.

Local factors

- **Skin lesions** – breaks in the skin are a breach in one of the body's first lines of defence against micro-organisms. Skin breaches and lesions are also a risk factor for colonisation with pathogenic micro-organisms such as meticillin resistant *Staphylococcus aureus* (MRSA) (Coia *et al.*, 2006). Chronic wounds, such as leg ulcers, can be colonised with bacteria including *Staphylococcus aureus, Streptococcus* spp. and *Pseudomonas aeruginosa* (McGuckin *et al.*, 2003). Traumatic wounds can often occur in unclean environments with the risk that micro-organisms can be introduced into the wound, for example tetanus from gardening accidents.

- **Ischaemia** – poor blood supply leads to a loss of nutrients to body tissues. This can lead to tissue necrosis, which provides an ideal environment for the colonisation and multiplication of anaerobic bacteria, such as *Clostridium tetani*, also known as gas gangrene. Inadequate blood supply can also lead to poor distribution of prophylactic antibiotics.

Invasive procedures

- **Cannulation** – peripheral, central venous and arterial catheters provide direct access for micro-organisms to enter the bloodstream. The presence of a cannula can lead to either local infection around the insertion site or life-threatening septicaemia.

- **Urinary catheterisation** – indwelling urinary catheters provide direct access for micro-organisms to access a patient's urinary system. In addition, constant urine draining bypasses the flushing action of urine that can help to expel micro-organisms during intermittent micturition. Biofilms that form in and on urinary catheters provide an ideal micro-environment in which pathogenic micro-organisms can migrate into the bladder and which can also protect micro-organisms from the actions of antibiotics (Spencer, 1999).

- **Intubation** – mechanical ventilation increases a patient's risk of pneumonia (Tablan *et al.*, 2003). Airway management procedures, such as suctioning, also increase risk of infection (Pierce, 1995).

- **Other invasive devices** – any invasive device breaching the skin provides an entry point for micro-organisms. Examples of other invasive devices include: chest drains, wound drains, intrathecal catheters and epidural catheters.

Drugs

- **Immunosuppressive drugs** – steroid therapy affects the body's inflammatory response processes; this is an important phase in the immune response to microbial invasion, which assists white blood cells in reaching the site of infection. Cytotoxic drugs used in chemotherapy can have a deleterious effect on cells of the immune system. Anti-rejection drugs used for transplant patients also suppress the body's immune function.

- **Antibiotics** – the administration of antibiotics can lead to the selection of antibiotic resistant bacteria in hospital patients (Cohen and Tartasky, 1997).

Disease

- **Diabetes mellitus** – is a risk factor for skin and soft tissue infection.

- **Renal disease** – patients on haemodialysis have a lowered immune function (Hörl, 1999). They are also at increased risk of infection if they have a vascular catheter in situ for dialysis purposes.

- **Immunodeficiency diseases** – conditions that affect the immune system, for example human immunodeficiency virus (HIV) or leukaemia are likely to increase a patient's risk of infection.

PROACTIVELY MANAGING INDIVIDUAL PATIENT RISK
Having assessed the risk factors that individual patients may have that increase the chance of their acquiring an infection, care and management strategies can be planned to minimise risk (Kingsley, 1992). Suggested strategies to address risks are detailed in Table 4.1.

ASSESSING RISK OF INFECTION TO OTHER PATIENTS
Risk of transmission of infection between patients varies depending on the micro-organism that is causing the infection, the route

Table 4.1 Suggested strategies for addressing individual patient infection risks.

Risk factor	Strategies for care and management
Age	• Consider appropriate placement for age group
Nutrition	• Undertake nutritional assessment • Ensure adequate nutrition provided during hospital stay • Consider nutritional supplements in consultation with dietetic staff
Restricted mobility	• Implement rehabilitation processes in consultation with physiotherapy and occupational therapy staff • Encourage passive exercises where appropriate • Consider patient positioning, for example an upward tilt on the bedhead as opposed to lying flat • Ensure adequate fluid intake to help prevent urinary stasis
Hygiene	• Apply standard infection control precautions to all patient contacts • Assess continence and implement appropriate continence care plans and use appropriate continence aids
Skin lesions	• Wound assessment and management • Avoid unnecessary wound exposure • Ensure wound covered with appropriate dressing • Aseptic technique for wound care • Awareness of signs and symptoms of infection and prompt action if evident • Adequate management of dermatological skin lesions (e.g. eczema or psoriasis) • Prevention of decubitus ulcers
Intravascular cannulae	• Remove as soon as no longer in use • Aseptic technique as minimum for all handling and access • Avoid unnecessary access points and interventions • Cover with sterile dressing • Daily assessment and documentation of insertion site condition • Change peripheral cannulae at 72 hours wherever possible
Urinary catheter	• Remove as soon as no longer in use • Aseptic technique for all handling • Ensure free drainage • Avoid disconnection of catheter from drainage bag • Securely anchor to prevent urethral trauma • Change catheter in accordance with manufacturers' instructions • Ensure adequate fluid intake
Intubation	• Elevation of the bed head • Clean/aseptic technique for suctioning • Use single use respiratory equipment or ensure adequate decontamination of reusable equipment
Patients with immune deficiency	• Boost levels of immunocompetency • Consider patient placement and environment • Compliance to standard infection control principles • Avoid contact with infectious staff or visitors through screening and occupational health policies

by which it is spread and the risk to other patients in that particular setting. To undertake a detailed risk assessment it is necessary to have knowledge of the source of the infection risk, how it is transmitted and what is likely to be contaminated (Kingsley, 1992). Chapter 14 details assessment of infection risk in relation to isolation.

Source of the infection risk

- **Respiratory tract** – coughs, sneezes, sore throats or cold like symptoms. Potential causative micro-organisms include *Mycobacterium tuberculosis*, respiratory syncytial virus or influenza.

- **Gastrointestinal tract** – diarrhoea and/or vomiting. Potential causative micro-organisms include norovirus, rotavirus, salmonella, campylobacter or hepatitis A.

- **Urinary tract** – frequency, dysuria, loin pain, offensive smell. Potential causative micro-organisms include *Klebsiella* spp., *Escherichia coli*.

- **Blood** – jaundice or hepatomegaly or no obvious signs and/or symptoms. Potential causative micro-organisms include HIV, hepatitis B or C.

- **Wound/skin** – signs and symptoms of infection include redness, pain, boils, pustules. There are many potential causative micro-organisms including *Staphylococcus aureus*.

Route of transmission

- Airborne
- Droplet
- Direct contact
- Indirect contact
- Percutaneous

What is the infective material?

- Respiratory secretions
- Nasopharyngeal secretions

- Faeces
- Vomit
- Blood
- Skin cells
- Exudate
- Pus

PROACTIVELY PREVENTING SPREAD OF INFECTION

Once an assessment has been made of the risk of transmission from an infected patient to other patients, the strategies in Table 4.2 can be considered to reduce the risk (Kingsley, 1992).

SCENARIO

Mr Stephens, a 78-year-old man, is admitted with acute urinary retention. He has an indwelling urethral catheter inserted to relieve this. He was recently in hospital for a minor surgical procedure but the wound has not completely healed. What are Mr Stephens' risk factors for infection and what should be done to reduce his risk of infection?

The presence of the urinary catheter presents a risk of urinary tract infection that could subsequently lead to bacteraemia. A plan of management for the urinary catheter should be put in place that includes aseptic technique for all handling and removal as soon as possible. The unhealed wound is also a risk factor for infection. The wound should be managed aseptically and assessed when dressings are performed for signs of infection. The wound should be kept covered at all times.

SUMMARY

Risk assessment is vital in informing nursing management and care strategies for patients at risk of infection as well as for preventing spread of infection from infected patients. For the patient at risk of infection the assessment focuses on general and local factors, invasive interventions, underlying diseases and medications. When assessing the risk of transmission from an infected patient, the assessment focuses on the source of infection, what is likely to be contaminated and how any contamination could be spread. Individual care plans can then be devised, focusing on the appropriate infection prevention strategies.

Table 4.2 Strategies to reduce the risk of transmission from an infected patient.

Source of infection	Infection transmission prevention strategies
Respiratory tract	• Advise on good respiratory hygiene • Consider need for isolation • Safe handling and disposal of respiratory secretions • Protective clothing as appropriate • Consider mask use, for example respirators for open pulmonary tuberculosis • Avoid aerosol generating activities in open ward area • Hand hygiene
Gastro-intestinal tract	• Consider need for isolation if diarrhoea uncontainable or patient vomiting • Dedicated toilet facilities or commode • Patient hand hygiene after toileting • Prompt cleaning/disinfection of spills • Gloves and aprons for handling vomit and faeces • Disposable bedpan or adequate disinfection of reusable bedpans • Hand hygiene
Urinary tract	• Consider need for isolation if multi-resistant micro-organism • Hand hygiene • Disposable receptacles for emptying or adequate disinfection of reusable receptacles • Prompt cleaning/disinfection of spills
Blood	• Standard precautions • Safe handling of sharps and prevention of needlestick injury • Hand hygiene • Prompt cleaning/disinfection of blood spills
Wound/skin	• Covering of wound with occlusive dressing where appropriate • Avoid exposure of wound where possible • Careful handling and disposal of wound dressing materials • Aseptic technique for dressing changes • Consider isolation of extensive skin infection or skin dispersal (e.g. infected eczema) • Hand hygiene

REFERENCES

Bowell, B. (1992) Assessing infection risks. *Nursing*, **4** (12), 19–23.

Cohen, F.L. and Tartasky, D. (1997) Microbial resistance to drug therapy: a review. *American Journal of Infection Control*, **25** (1), 51–64.

Coia, J.E., Duckworth, G.K., Edwards, D.I. *et al.* (2006) Guidelines for the control and prevention of meticillin resistant *Staphylococcus aureus* (MRSA) in healthcare facilities. *Journal of Hospital Infection*, **63** (suppl.) s1–44.

Hörl, W.H. (1999) Neutrophil function and infections in uremia. *American Journal of Kidney Disease*, **33**, xiv–xxii.

Kingsley, A. (1992) First step towards a desired outcome. Preventing infection by risk recognition. *Professional Nurse*, **7** (11), 725–729.

Malone, D.L., Genuit, T., Tracy, J.K., Gannon, C. and Napolitano, L. M. (2002) Surgical site infection: re-analysis of risk factors. *Journal of Surgical Research*, **103** (1), 89–95.

McGuckin, M., Goldman, R., Bolton, L. and Salcido, R. (2003) The clinical relevance of microbiology in acute and chronic wounds. *Advances in Skin and Wound Care*, **16** (1), 12–23.

Pierce, L. (1995) *Guide to Mechanical Ventilation and Respiratory Care.* W.B. Saunders Company, Philadelphia.

Pratt, R., Morgan, S., Hughes, J. *et al.* (2002) Healthcare governance and the modernisation of the NHS: infection prevention and control. *British Journal of Infection Control*, **3** (5), 16–25.

Spencer, R.C.S. (1999) Novel methods for the prevention of infection of intravascular devices. *Journal of Hospital Infection*, **43** (suppl.), S127–135.

Tablan, O.C., Anderson, L.J., Besser, R., Bridges, C. and Hajjeh, R. (2003) *Guidelines for Preventing Healthcare Associated Pneumonia.* Available at: www.cdc.gov (accessed 20 November 2006).

Wilkie, M.H., Almond, M.K. and Marsh, F.P. (1992) Diagnosis and management of urinary tract infection in adults. *British Medical Journal*, **305**, 1137–1141.

5 | Standard Infection Control Principles

INTRODUCTION

Standard infection control principles should be applied to the care of all patients, regardless of their infection status. These principles are aimed at preventing infection both to patients and to healthcare workers. This chapter covers the essential principles of infection prevention that can be applied in all hospital settings.

LEARNING OBJECTIVES

By the end of this chapter you will be able to:

❏ Define the terms 'universal precautions' and 'standard precautions'
❏ Describe effective hand decontamination techniques
❏ Identify appropriate protective clothing for use in clinical settings
❏ Describe how to prevent contamination incidents
❏ Identify key environmental aspects of standard precautions

UNIVERSAL AND STANDARD PRECAUTIONS

Universal infection control precautions developed in the 1980s, largely in response to concerns over blood borne viruses, including hepatitis B and human immunodeficiency virus (HIV). Prior to this time, precautions had mainly been based around assessment of risk according to a patient's infection status. The long incubation period and potential carrier status for some blood borne viruses meant that a number of patients who had these infections were not identified and therefore the correct precautions were not taken. In addition, there was discrimination attached to the risk assessment and some patients were treated as potentially infectious due to their lifestyle, for example gay men. Universal precautions were introduced to remove this discrimination, to reduce the risk from patients in the incubation or carrier phase of disease and to protect the healthcare worker. The risk assessment in universal precautions is based on the risk of contact with blood or the body fluids with highest concentration of virus. The following body fluids should be handled with the same precautions as blood:

- Cerebrospinal fluid
- Amniotic fluid
- Synovial fluid
- Peritoneal fluid
- Vaginal fluid
- Semen
- Breast milk
- Pleural fluid
- Pericardial fluid
- Saliva in association with dentistry
- Any other body fluid visibly contaminated with blood
- Unfixed tissues and organs (United Kingdom Health Departments, 1998)

Whilst universal precautions are appropriate principles for prevention of blood borne viruses, the risk of infection from other body fluids, for example pseudomonas in sputum, is not addressed, and neither is prevention of risk of infection from one patient to another. To address this, practice in both the UK and the US has moved to standard precautions. This is a set of standard infection control principles that should be applied to the care of all patients undergoing healthcare and includes all activities where there is a risk of contact with blood, body fluids, excretions and secretions. These principles include: hand hygiene; use of protective clothing; safe handling and disposal of sharps; and environmental hygiene (Pratt *et al.*, 2007).

HAND HYGIENE

Hand hygiene is considered to be one of the most important infection prevention measures. Micro-organisms found on hands fall into two categories.

Resident organisms
These organisms are deeply seated within the epidermis and are not readily removable. They are not generally associated with transmission of infection in hospitals. Resident micro-organisms include coagulase negative staphylococci and diptheroids.

Transient organisms
These organisms are found on the skin surface and also beneath the superficial layers of the stratum corneum. They generally transfer to healthcare workers' hands through contact with people or equipment. They can be easily transferred from a healthcare worker's hands to a patient or an item of equipment, hence the term transient. Transient organisms can be viral, bacterial or fungal and can include *Staphylococcus aureus*, *Candida* spp., respiratory syncytial virus.

ASSESSMENT OF HAND DECONTAMINATION NEEDS
Hand hygiene needs are based on an assessment of four key factors:

- The level of anticipated contact with patients
- The extent of contamination that may occur with that contact
- The patient care activities being performed
- The susceptibility of the patient (Pratt *et al.*, 2007)

When to decontaminate hands
Hands should be decontaminated before and after each and every episode of direct patient care (Pratt *et al.*, 2007). In addition, hands should be decontaminated after any activity or contact that potentially results in hands becoming contaminated. The following list gives examples of when hands should be decontaminated, but is not exhaustive:

- Before commencing and leaving duty or a work area
- Before preparing, handling and eating food
- Before and after handling any invasive device in a patient
- Before and after administering medications
- After handling used linen (i.e. bedmaking)

- Before and after an aseptic technique
- Before any direct patient care and contact
- When moving from a 'dirty' to a 'clean' activity on the same patient
- After handling contaminated waste
- After handling contaminated equipment

Which method of hand decontamination to use

For hand hygiene on a ward, generally routine hand hygiene, to remove transient micro-organisms is sufficient. For certain procedures, for example insertion of a central venous line, surgical hand hygiene to remove transient micro-organisms and to reduce levels of resident micro-organisms is necessary. Surgical hand hygiene is described in detail in Chapter 12.

Hands that are visibly soiled or are heavily contaminated with dirt or organic matter should be washed with liquid soap and water (Pratt *et al.*, 2007). In most circumstances a general liquid soap, that has detergent but no antimicrobial properties, is sufficient. Antiseptic solutions, such as chlorhexidine gluconate, povidone iodine or triclosan may be needed for hand hygiene in certain circumstances, for example in the care of immunocompromised patients. Alcohol based hand gels are a useful method of hand decontamination and are now considered the preferred method for routine hand hygiene (WHO, 2005). However, alcohol based hand gels may be less effective against some viruses that cause gastroenteritis and *Clostridium difficile* spores. Hand washing with soap and water is preferable if a patient has diarrhoea due to one of these causes. The following flow chart (Figure 5.1) is useful in determining which method of hand hygiene to use.

HAND HYGIENE TECHNIQUE

Even if hands are decontaminated each and every time needed, if hands are not decontaminated effectively there is still a risk of transmission of infection. When decontaminating hands the thumbs and tips of fingers are areas that are very commonly missed (Taylor, 1978). A good hand hygiene technique must ensure that all areas of the hands are adequately decontaminated.

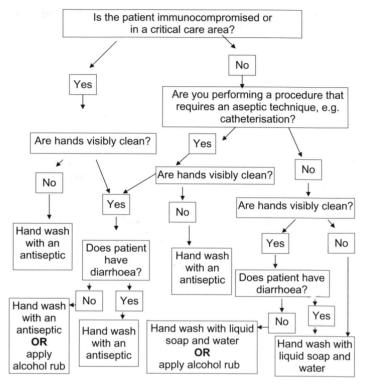

Figure 5.1 Flow chart for hand hygiene.

The presence of stoned rings and watches or wrist jewellery can impede good hand hygiene (Infection Control Nurses Association, 2002a). Nails should be kept short, as many micro-organisms are harboured beneath them (Larson, 1989). Artificial nails and nail jewellery or art should not be worn for the same reason.

Hands should be dried using good quality paper towels, taking care not to recontaminate hands when disposing of the paper towel. Hot air hand dryers should not be used in clinical settings as hand dryers are not as effective in removing bacteria from hands as paper towels and may themselves be contaminated with pathogenic bacteria (Blackmore, 1989).

Procedure for hand washing

- Remove all wrist and hand jewellery.
- Cover cuts and abrasions with waterproof dressings.
- Prepare hands by wetting under tepid running water.
- Apply liquid soap or antiseptic preparation.
- Ensuring hand wash solution comes into contact with all the surfaces of the hands and wrists, rub hands vigorously together for 10–15 seconds; pay particular attention to the tips of fingers, the thumbs and the areas between the fingers.
- Rinse hands thoroughly under running water.
- Dry hands carefully but thoroughly with paper hand towel. (Pratt *et al.*, 2007; Health Protection Scotland, 2006a)

Figure 5.2 shows the six-step hand washing technique devised by Ayliffe *et al.* (1978) to ensure all areas of the hands are covered.

Procedure for application of alcohol hand gel

- Only use if hands are not contaminated with organic matter or body fluids.
- Apply sufficient hand gel to palm of the first hand.
- Press the fingertips of the second hand into the dispensed gel in the palm of the first hand.
- Tip the alcohol from the first hand into the palm of the second hand.
- Press the fingertips of the first hand into the gel in the palm of the second hand.
- Spread the alcohol gel over the surfaces of both hands.
- Spread the alcohol gel over both hands until it has evaporated.

HAND CARE
There is some evidence to suggest that the resident micro-organisms on hands can be altered if skin is damaged, which can

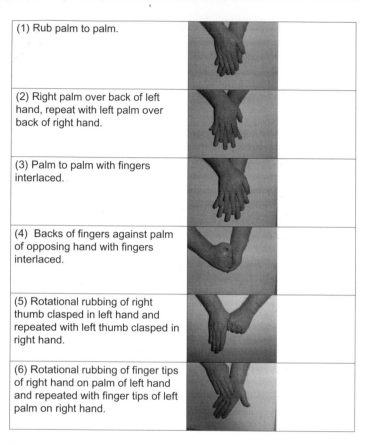

(1) Rub palm to palm.	
(2) Right palm over back of left hand, repeat with left palm over back of right hand.	
(3) Palm to palm with fingers interlaced.	
(4) Backs of fingers against palm of opposing hand with fingers interlaced.	
(5) Rotational rubbing of right thumb clasped in left hand and repeated with left thumb clasped in right hand.	
(6) Rotational rubbing of finger tips of right hand on palm of left hand and repeated with finger tips of left palm on right hand.	

Figure 5.2 Six-step hand hygiene technique (after Ayliffe *et al.*, 1978).

then lead to greater hand carriage of micro-organisms responsible for hospital acquired infections (Kownatzki, 2003). To protect the integrity of hands, thorough rinsing and drying is important when hand washing. Hand creams containing an emollient are useful for maintaining skin integrity and hydration (Pratt *et al.*, 2007). They need not be applied constantly during a shift but should be used when taking breaks and when leaving a shift of duty. It is preferable to use specifically designed hand cream dispensers as communal jars of hand cream may become contaminated with micro-organisms (Gould, 1994). Staff who suffer ongoing hand lesions should consult their occupational health department for assessment.

HAND HYGIENE AND PATIENTS

Patients should be involved in hand hygiene both to ensure that they are able to decontaminate their hands when needed and in helping to improve hand hygiene compliance of healthcare workers. Patients should always be offered, and encouraged to use, hand hygiene facilities prior to eating and after using toilet facilities. If it is not possible for patients to use a hand washing sink they can be offered hand wipes or alcohol gel. Individually wrapped hand wipes can be placed on patients' meal trays to encourage hand hygiene prior to eating and drinking.

Patients and visitors should also be encouraged to ask healthcare workers if they have decontaminated their hands before they have contact with them. This patient empowerment has been found to be effective in improving hand hygiene compliance (McGuckin *et al.*, 2001).

IMPROVING HAND HYGIENE COMPLIANCE

Although hand hygiene is recognised as an important factor in prevention of hospital acquired infections, there is good evidence that healthcare workers do not decontaminate their hands as often or as effectively as they should (e.g. Perry and Gore, 1997). The following list is not exhaustive but is useful in improving compliance:

- The provision of sufficient hand hygiene sinks that are conveniently located in clinical areas
- The provision of alcohol hand gel either located at the point of patient contact or carried by staff
- Patient challenge to staff
- Staff challenge to colleagues
- Role models in good hand hygiene amongst all disciplines of healthcare workers
- Monitoring and feedback of hand hygiene compliance

- Clear hand hygiene policies and procedures
- Posters reminding staff about the importance of hand hygiene and appropriate techniques, which are regularly changed or rotated

PROTECTIVE CLOTHING – GLOVES

Gloves are an important feature of standard and universal precautions and as personal protective equipment are subject to requirements under the Control of Substances Hazardous to Health (COSHH) Regulations (HSE, 1999) in that they must be fit for the purpose intended. Gloves are worn in healthcare for the following reasons:

- To protect the healthcare worker from contact with blood and body fluids
- To protect the healthcare worker from contact with hazardous chemicals and substances, for example disinfectants or chemotherapeutic agents
- To reduce risk of cross infection by preventing staff hands becoming contaminated with micro-organisms from patients and vice versa

Whether gloves need to be worn and the type of glove to be worn is based on a risk assessment. This risk can be assessed using the following prompts:

- Is the risk of infection to the patient or to the healthcare worker?
- Does the activity being carried out require sterile or non-sterile gloves to be worn?
- What is the likely extent of contact with blood, body fluids, secretions and excretions?
- What contact is likely with non-intact skin or mucous membranes? (Pratt *et al.*, 2007)

CHOOSING THE RIGHT GLOVE

There are a variety of glove materials available in healthcare. Natural rubber latex is still currently considered to be the glove material of choice due to its protective ability (Pratt *et al.*, 2007).

Other synthetic glove materials are available that may provide similar protective properties to latex. Table 5.1 details the properties of different types of gloves.

Table 5.2 gives examples of clinical activities and the types of gloves that should be considered.

Whichever glove type is used, the following principles also apply:

Table 5.1 Glove properties (Infection Control Nurses Association, 2002b).

Glove type	Properties
Natural rubber latex	• Flexible and durable • Close fitting • Generally comfortable to wear • Good tactile sensitivity • Little impairment on dexterity • Higher tensile strength • Lower leakage rates than vinyl
Vinyl	• Possibly less effective viral barrier than latex • Lower tensile strength than latex • Prone to leakage • Inelastic and less close fitting than latex • No documented allergenic reactions to date • Suitable for latex free environment
Nitrile	• Excellent biological barrier • Less elastic than latex • Can be used for some chemicals • Suitable for latex free environments
Tactylon	• Similar physical properties to latex • Less susceptible to degradation than latex • Rapidly breaks down in contact with some chemicals • Suitable for latex free environments
Polychloroprene	• Effective biological barrier • Resists permeability from some chemicals • Similar elasticity to latex • Suitable for latex free environment
Polythene	• Ill-fitting • Heat sealed seams prone to splitting • Tendency to tear • Not recommended in clinical settings

Table 5.2 Examples of healthcare activities with appropriate gloves to use.

Activity	Type of glove to use
Surgical procedure	• Sterile latex surgeons • Sterile neoprene surgeons • Sterile tactylon • Sterile nitrile surgeons
Aseptic procedure where risk of exposure to blood or bloodstained body fluid is likely (e.g. accessing a central venous line)	• Sterile latex examination • Sterile nitrile examination • Sterile neoprene examination
Non-aseptic procedures where: • Exposure to blood or bloodstained body fluid is likely (e.g. emptying a catheter bag of a patient with haematuria) • The glove is likely to be subject to pressure, pulling or twisting • A close fitting glove and tactile sensitivity is required • Handling of sharps is involved Decontamination tasks with chemical disinfectants	• Non-sterile latex examination • Non-sterile nitrile examination • Non-sterile neoprene examination
Aseptic procedures where exposure to blood or bloodstained body fluid is unlikely (e.g. simple wound dressing)	• Sterile vinyl examination
Non-aseptic procedures where exposure to blood or bloodstained body fluid is unlikely (e.g. emptying a stoma bag) Cleaning with detergent and water	• Non-sterile vinyl examination
Food handling	• Non-sterile vinyl examination • Non-sterile polythene examination

- Hands should be decontaminated before wearing gloves for all aseptic procedures.
- Gloves should be removed immediately a task has been completed (Health Protection Scotland, 2006b); observational studies have demonstrated environmental contamination through not removing gloves and handling inanimate objects such as telephones and infusion devices (Girou *et al.*, 2004).

- Hands should always be decontaminated after removal of gloves; gloves can leak during use and hands can become contaminated when removing gloves (Pratt *et al.*, 2007).
- Gloves should be changed between different care activities on the same patient.
- The correct size glove should be worn; incorrectly fitting gloves can lead to dexterity problems, skin irritation and finger muscle fatigue with prolonged use (Infection Control Nurses Association, 2002b).
- Only powder free gloves should be used in healthcare.
- Gloves should be low in residual accelerators and protein.
- Do not wear gloves for longer than is necessary; excess wearing can cause air occlusion and excess moisture, leading to skin breakdown and providing an ideal environment in which some micro-organisms can thrive (Truscott, 1995).
- Gloves are a single use item; they should not be decontaminated by washing or alcohol gel as this can affect their integrity, performance and effectiveness, reducing their ability to provide a protective barrier (Infection Control Nurses Association, 2002b).
- Used gloves should be disposed of as clinical waste (Pratt *et al.*, 2007).
- Always consider risk of latex allergy before using latex gloves.

LATEX ALLERGIES
Repeated exposure to latex carries a risk of latex allergy and concerns over allergies amongst healthcare workers is increasing (Medical Devices Agency, 1996). Risk assessment for latex allergy in both the healthcare worker and the patient is important when choosing which glove to wear. Risk of latex allergy is greater in the following individuals:

- Healthcare workers with repeated and prolonged exposure to latex (e.g. those working in operating theatres or dentistry)
- Atopic individuals who have a predisposition to produce immunogloblin E when exposed to an allergen; this can include individuals with eczema, hayfever and asthma
- Individuals with the following food allergies (Medical Devices Agency, 1996):

— Banana
— Kiwi fruit
— Chestnuts
— Avocado
— Passion fruit
— Tomato
— Potato
— Star fruit

• Patients who have undergone repeated healthcare interventions, including patients with the following conditions (Infection Control Nurses Association, 2002b):

— Spina bifida
— Myelodysplasia
— Chronic bowel and bladder dysfunction

Latex allergy manifests itself in two distinct patterns:

Type I Symptoms are relatively immediate and occur within 5–30 minutes of exposure. Reactions range from skin redness, wheezing, to life threatening anaphylaxis. This type of reaction is due to exposure to the natural proteins in the latex.

Type IV Symptoms are less immediate and occur within 6–48 hours of exposure. This type of allergy usually manifests as a skin rash or contact dermatitis. The reaction is due to chemical accelerators used in the manufacturing process.

PROTECTIVE CLOTHING – APRONS AND GOWNS

Aprons and gowns are worn to protect healthcare workers' clothing from contamination with blood and body fluids (Infection Control Nurses Association, 2002b) as well as to protect patients from infection when they are undergoing procedures such as insertion of a central venous catheter, when a sterile gown will be worn. The type of apron or gown to be worn depends on an assessment of the risk of contact with body fluids. A plastic apron will protect the area of a uniform most commonly contaminated (Babb *et al.*, 1983). If extensive contact with blood or bloodstained fluid is likely, for example when caring for a patient with multiple trauma, then a long sleeved, fluid repellent gown should be worn. Sterile gowns are worn for some invasive and for all surgical procedures.

Use of plastic disposable aprons

- Worn when there is a risk of body fluid splash to uniforms
- Worn to protect uniforms from micro-organisms when caring for patients requiring isolation precautions
- May be worn when carrying out aseptic procedures, such as wound dressings; aprons used for this purpose must be kept in a clean environment as contamination may occur if stored in dirty utility areas (Callaghan, 1998)
- Are single use and should be discarded after each episode of care or task
- May be worn for decontamination activities, including cleaning and disinfection
- Discard as clinical waste

Use of long sleeved gowns

- Worn where there is a risk of extensive contamination of uniform or clothing
- Worn for certain procedures on patients requiring isolation precautions, for example airway management of a patient with pandemic influenza
- Must be fluid repellent
- Must be single use and discarded after each episode of care or task
- Discard as clinical waste

PROTECTIVE CLOTHING – MASKS AND RESPIRATORS

Face-masks should be worn when there is a risk of blood, body fluid or other secretion to the face or mouth (Pratt *et al.*, 2007). Where there is a need to protect healthcare workers from micro-organisms spread by the airborne route, then respiratory protective equipment that provides an appropriate level of filtration is required (Pratt *et al.*, 2007). Masks are rarely worn in wards or departments for general care, but may be required in exceptional circumstances, for example when caring for a patient with a massive haematemesis. Surgical masks should be worn when carrying out airway management on a patient with meningococcal meningitis (Public Health Laboratory Service, 2002). Respirators are recommended when caring for patients with certain infectious respiratory diseases, including infectious tuberculosis (The Interdepartmental Working Group on Tuberculosis, 1998), Avian influenza (Health Protection Agency, 2004) and for aerosol generating activities in pandemic influenza (Department of Health, 2005).

The difference between masks and respirators
Face-masks are generally worn to prevent the wearer from expelling droplets into the environment and if fluid resistant, to protect the wearer from splashes. Respirators are made to specific standards; EN149:2001 FFP3 in the UK and Europe and NIOSH-approved in the US. Respirators may have a breathing valve on them or may be manufactured without; the presence of a valve does not indicate a higher level of filtration. EN149:2001 FFP3 respirators provide the highest level of protection. EN149:2001 FFP2 respirators provide a lower level of protection; these are equivalent to the US graded N95 respirators. Figure 5.3 shows a surgical mask, an FFP2 and an FFP3 respirator.

Wearing a respirator
Where respiratory protection is being worn to protect healthcare workers from airborne infection, it is important that they fit correctly, with no air entry around the sides. The respirator should be a snug fit over the face. The strings or elastic ties should be positioned, one at the top of the head and one at the base of the neck to keep the respirator firmly in place over the nose and chin. The metal or plastic strip should be across the nose and this should be moulded to the shape of the bridge of the nose to provide a snug fit. Formal testing of how well the respirator fits is required in certain circumstances but a quick check of fit can be performed by panting hard a few times; if the respirator is fitting correctly it should move in and out as you breathe.

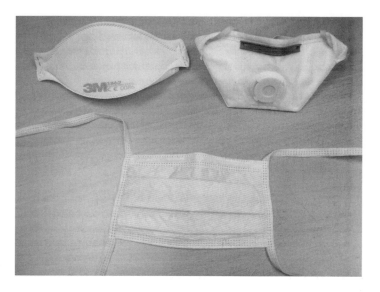

Figure 5.3 Different types of masks and respirators. From top left clockwise FFP2 respirator, FFP3 respirator with value, surgical face mask with fluid shield.

Most respirators will give protection for up to eight hours when worn continuously. If they are removed from the nose and chin they should be discarded and not used again. Respirators should be removed by holding the strings only, taking care not to touch the outside with the hands, and discarded as clinical waste.

PROTECTIVE CLOTHING – EYE PROTECTION
Eye protection is worn when there is a risk of blood, body fluid, secretions or excretions to the eyes (Pratt *et al.*, 2007). Eye protection may be in the form of goggles or a visor attached to a surgical mask.

USE AND DISPOSAL OF SHARPS
Sharp instruments and items are commonly used throughout hospital care. In the UK, injuries from sharps account for approximately 17% of all reported injuries to healthcare workers (National

Audit Office, 2003). The major risk from sharps injuries is blood borne viruses; however, other infections may be transmitted in this manner, for example a needlestick injury during the taking of a catheter specimen of urine could result in bacterial infection to a healthcare worker if there are bacteria present in the urine. The relative risks if a health care worker has a needlestick injury from a patient known to have a blood borne virus are:

Hepatitis B	33% (1 in 3)
Hepatitis C	1–3% (1 in 10–30)
Human immunodeficiency virus	0.3% (1 in 300)

The risk of disease if the injury to a healthcare worker is from splash of blood or bloodstained body fluid to mucous membranes is reduced by one third.

Principles for safe use of sharps

Up to 40% of sharps injuries occur during the actual use of a sharp and before disposal (Infection Control Nurses Association, 2003). Prevention of sharps injuries starts before the point of use and should be based on the following principles (UK Health Departments, 1998; Pratt *et al.*, 2007; Health Protection Scotland, 2006c):

- Avoid the use of sharps wherever possible.
- Never carry sharps by hand; always use an appropriate receptacle.
- Carry out a risk assessment before starting a procedure involving a sharp; if the patient is uncooperative seek assistance.
- Take a sharps bin to the bedside for immediate disposal as opposed to carrying a used sharp across a clinical area.
- Do not re-sheath or bend needles wherever possible.
- If re-sheathing is necessary, for example during dental procedures, a re-sheathing device should be used or the following one-handed scoop technique used (see Figure 5.4):

    — Place the sheath on a flat surface
    — Slide the needle in from the side
    — When the needle tip is fully covered, re-sheathing can be completed by hand

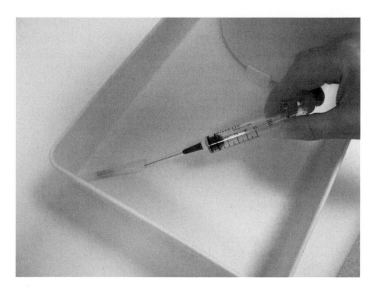

Figure 5.4 Scoop re-sheathing technique.

- Wear the appropriate protective clothing, such as gloves; this may not stop the needle penetrating but may reduce the amount of blood that is inoculated and therefore reduce risk of blood borne virus infection.
- Do not disassemble needles prior to disposal.
- Use safety devices where available.
- Remove needles from syringes before transporting for blood gas analysis, and similar procedures, and replace with a blind hub.

Principles for safe disposal of sharps
Up to 35% of sharps injuries occur during disposal (Infection Control Nurses Association, 2003). The following principles should be applied to disposal and to use of sharps bins:

- The user of a sharp is responsible for safe disposal.
- Only sharps bins that are United Nations approved should be used for disposal of sharps (HSE, 1999).

- Sharps bins should be assembled correctly prior to use and the appropriate information entered on the sharps bin label.
- Bins must never be filled above the fill line indicated on all sharps containers; it is the responsibility of all users to seal a bin when this line is reached.
- Sharps bins should be used for the disposal of sharps waste only wherever possible.
- Sharps bins should be located at a suitable height, never on the floor or above shoulder level.
- Wherever possible brackets should be used to secure sharps bins.
- Sharps bins must be located out of access by the general public.
- The temporary closure on the bin should be used to prevent accidental access to the bin between use.
- Once the fill line has been reached, the lid should be fully closed and locked.
- Filled sharps bins should be labelled and tagged with the ward/department, hospital, date of disposal and the signature of the person disposing.
- Filled sharps bins awaiting collection should be kept in a safe place.
- Staff transporting filled sharps bins should wear suitable protective clothing and avoid carrying the bin close to their body.

MANAGEMENT OF SHARPS INJURIES

Prompt management of sharps injuries is important to enable a risk assessment and appropriate action to be taken. Reporting of sharps injuries is also important in order to identify trends in injuries that may be addressed by the introduction of safer devices or techniques. Other contamination injuries require the same actions as sharps injuries, for example blood splash to eyes or mouth. The generic term 'contamination incident' is often used when referring to needlestick and splash injuries. Figure 5.5 details the initial actions that should be followed in event of a contamination incident.

After these initial actions a risk assessment will be undertaken and the following actions will be taken where appropriate:

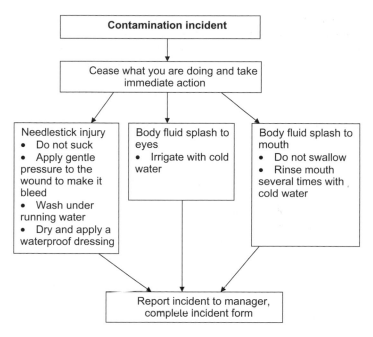

Figure 5.5 Action in event of contamination incident to staff.

- If the source patient is known they will be counselled and if in agreement their blood will be tested for hepatitis B, hepatitis C and human immunodeficiency virus (HIV).
- The injured healthcare worker's blood will be taken and stored.
- If the risk of HIV infection is thought to be sufficiently high, post-exposure prophylaxis will be offered to the injured healthcare worker.
- If the healthcare worker is not immune to hepatitis B, passive immunity in the form of immunoglobulin or active immunity in the form of an accelerated course of hepatitis B vaccination will be considered.
- Occupational health departments will counsel the healthcare worker in terms of work activities, safe sex and blood donation during the follow-up period.

- Occupational health departments will arrange future testing of the healthcare worker where appropriate.

Occasionally patients can experience contamination incidents from healthcare workers or other patients. The following are examples of such injuries:

- A needlestick injury occurring during an operation where the injured healthcare worker bleeds into the patient's tissues
- The feeding of breast milk to the wrong baby
- A patient injured from a needle accidentally discarded on the floor

These injuries should be followed up in the same manner as injuries to healthcare workers, but they are often managed by infection control teams as opposed to occupational health teams.

WASTE

Healthcare generates many different types of waste. Under the Environmental Protection Act and Controlled Waste Regulations (DoE, 1991) hospitals are required by law to dispose of waste correctly. Nurses play an important role in this by ensuring that they segregate waste correctly as they dispose of it.

Clinical waste is defined as waste that arises from healthcare practice that could cause infection to persons coming into contact with it. Clinical waste also includes any waste that consists partly or wholly of body tissue, blood, body excretions, swabs or dressings (DoE, 1991). Under the Hazardous Waste Regulations (2005) infectious waste is described as that containing viable micro-organisms or their toxins that are known or reliably believed to cause disease in man or other living organisms. Current waste regulations require that infectious clinical waste be disposed of in containers that are largely yellow in colour. The following principles should be applied to the handling and disposal of clinical waste in wards and departments (UK Health Departments, 1998; Health Protection Scotland, 2006d; DoH, 2006):

- Waste should be disposed of promptly into the correct receptacle.
- Clinical waste should be segregated from other wastes at the point of disposal and at all stages of the waste disposal process.
- Nurses handling clinical waste should wear protective clothing based on a risk assessment of likely contamination.
- Clinical waste bins should have foot operating lids so that waste can be disposed of without touching the lid.
- Waste bags should not be over filled; they should be replaced before they become too full for the bag to be securely sealed to prevent leakage.
- Receptacles containing liquid clinical waste may require disposal in rigid leak-proof clinical waste bins.
- Clinical waste must be labelled with the source of the waste to enable it to be traced back to the producer in event of a spill or inappropriate disposal.
- Clinical waste awaiting collection must be stored securely away from members of the public.

LINEN HANDLING

Linen has rarely been associated with outbreaks of infection; however, there have been reports of infections when linen has been inadequately laundered locally rather than in a commercial or dedicated laundry facility. A *Streptococcus pyogenes* outbreak in a neonatal unit was traced back to a unit based washing machine (Telfer-Brunton, 1995) and an outbreak of *Acinetobacter* was linked to inadequate laundry processes for pillows (Weernink *et al.*, 1995).

Used linen that is being sent to a hospital laundry facility is colour coded in accordance with national policy (DoH, 1995) to enable laundry workers to use the correct washing process.

Used linen is linen that has been used within the hospital but is not visibly contaminated with blood, body fluids or from a patient who is being isolated for an infectious condition. This type of linen is usually placed in a white bag made of either material or plastic.

Soiled/foul linen is linen that has been used and is contaminated with body fluids such as urine or faeces. This type of linen is usually placed in a white or clear plastic bag that should be tied before being placed in an outer white bag of the same type as for used linen.

Infected linen is linen that is heavily soiled with blood, body fluids containing highly transmissible micro-organisms, or is from patients who are in isolation for an infectious disease. This type of linen is placed in a red dissolvable bag, which is tied, and then is placed in a red outer bag made of linen or plastic. This linen is not washed in the same way as soiled or used linen. Instead it is usually washed in a separate machine. The laundry workers do not handle the linen; it is placed in the washing machine inside the red dissolvable bag, which then dissolves during the wash process.

Other types of linen are sometimes segregated into different coloured bags, for example staff clothing including scrubs, clean damaged linen for repair. The colour coding for this is often determined at local level and hospital policy should be followed.

Principles for safe handling of linen

- Clean linen should be stored in a manner that protects it from dust, preferably in a cupboard or container with the door kept closed.
- Clean linen should not be placed on potentially contaminated surfaces, for example toilet seats, bin lids or linen skip lids.
- Clean linen, if dropped onto the floor, should be re-laundered as the floor is one of the ward areas most heavily contaminated with micro-organisms.
- Care should be taken when making beds not to shake linen to minimise the amount of dust created.
- Used, soiled or infected linen should not be carried through ward areas, as skin scales and micro-organisms can be shed into the environment whilst it is being carried; a linen skip should be taken to the bedside and the linen discarded there.

- Used, soiled or infected linen should not be placed on the floor before disposal.
- Aprons may need to be worn to protect uniforms from contamination.
- Gloves and aprons should be worn when handling soiled/ fouled and infected linen.
- Hands should always be decontaminated after handling used, soiled and infected linen as well as after handling linen skips. (Health Protection Scotland, 2006e)

Local laundry facilities

It is preferable for all hospital laundry to be processed in a dedicated laundry facility. Occasionally it may be necessary to have local laundry facilities. In these circumstances the following principles should be applied (Infection Control Nurses Association, 2004):

- Washing machines must be located in a designated, appropriate area that has easily cleanable surfaces.
- The washing machine must be on a pre-planned maintenance schedule.
- The laundry room must have a hand wash basin.
- Patients' own laundry must be segregated and washed in individual batches.
- The maximum wash code for the laundry must be used.
- Contaminated laundry should not be washed by hand before placing in the washing machine.
- Linen should be tumble dried using a dryer exhausted to the outside wherever possible.
- Wet linen must not be hung to dry in sluice rooms, bathrooms or ward areas.

Uniforms

Uniforms are not classified as protective clothing as they are worn to identify the wearer rather than to protect them from microorganisms. Uniforms have been found to be contaminated before and after a spell of duty (Callaghan, 1998; Perry *et al.*, 2001). Nursing staff should wear a clean uniform daily and should wear protective clothing appropriately to prevent risk of contamination. Where laundry facilities are available nursing staff should use these. If laundering uniforms at home the following principles should be applied:

- Launder uniforms separately to any other clothing.
- Launder on the maximum temperature the material will allow, preferably at a minimum of 60°C.
- Tumble dry and/or iron uniforms to further reduce levels of micro-organisms.
- Store clean uniforms in a manner that protects them from contamination, for example covered in a wardrobe.
- Transport clean uniforms to work in a manner that protects them from contamination, for example in a plastic bag. (Callaghan, 1998; Perry *et al.*, 2001; Royal College of Nursing, undated)

ENVIRONMENTAL CLEANLINESS
Outbreaks of infection have been linked to microbial contamination in the clinical environment (e.g. Rampling *et al.*, 2001). Hospital premises should be maintained visibly clean and dust free; no soiling should be evident and it should be acceptable in the eyes of patients and visitors (Pratt *et al.*, 2007). Items of equipment have also been found to be contaminated with micro-organisms (e.g. enterococci and *Staphylococcus aureus*) and have been linked to outbreaks of infection, for example blood pressure cuffs and *Clostridium difficile* (Manian *et al.*, 1996). Environmental and equipment decontamination is covered in detail in Chapter 16.

SPILLS OF BLOOD AND BODY FLUIDS
Any spills of blood and body fluids should be cleared up promptly, not only from an infection control perspective, but to reduce risk of slips and falls. To comply with health and safety requirements, nurses have a duty to take action and deal with any spills they are made aware of. Local policies should detail clearly who has responsibility for managing spills of body fluids; where nursing staff are not required to clear the spill they have a duty to make the area safe by alerting the appropriate person to manage the spill and alerting others to the risk of slip, for example by the use of a wet floor sign.

National guidance currently recommends the use of a chlorine based disinfectant for clearing of blood spills (UK Health Departments, 1998). In some hospitals it is policy to use a detergent only; where this is in place hospital policy should be followed.

Procedure for small spills of blood or body fluids

- Ensure area is well ventilated.
- Cover spill with chlorine releasing granules.
- Leave for two minutes.
- Wearing gloves, use disposable paper cloth or towels to pick up granules and dispose into clinical waste.
- Remove gloves and decontaminate hands.
- Ensure area is cleaned with detergent and water.

Procedure for large spills of blood or body fluids

- Ensure area is well ventilated.
- Cover spill with disposable paper cloths or towels.
- Pour a solution of 10000 ppm sodium hypochlorite (e.g. Haztabs or Milton) onto the paper towels covering the spill.
- Leave for two minutes.
- Wearing gloves, remove disposable paper, ensuring the spill is removed.
- Dispose into clinical waste.
- Remove gloves and decontaminate hands.
- Ensure area is cleaned with detergent and water.

Procedure for spills of blood or body fluids on carpets and soft furnishing and for spills of urine

Chlorine may bleach carpets and soft furnishing and should therefore not be used for spills. Urine in combination with chlorine may be hazardous; therefore chlorine should not be used on urine spills. The following procedure should be followed:

- Wearing gloves, clear spill using disposable paper cloth or towel.
- Dispose into clinical waste.
- Remove gloves and decontaminate hands.
- Clean area of spill with detergent and water.

SCENARIO

Mr Thomas is a 56-year-old male, known to be a carrier of hepatitis C, who is admitted to a surgical ward for a planned large bowel resection. What protective clothing would you wear for carrying out nursing care activities?

Gloves would only need to be worn for procedures where contact with blood or body fluids was possible, for example emptying a urinary catheter bag. A plastic apron would be worn for activities where uniform could become contaminated with body fluids or micro-organisms, for example bedmaking. Masks would not normally be needed for procedures carried out in the ward. Eye protection would only be needed if there was a risk of the nurse's eyes being splashed with blood or body fluids. This is unlikely with most procedures carried out in the ward.

SUMMARY

Standard infection control precautions are applied to the care of all patients in hospital to prevent the spread of infection to staff and to other patients, based on a risk assessment of the healthcare activity being performed. The key components of standard precautions are:

(1) Hand hygiene
(2) Protective clothing
(3) Decontamination of equipment and the environment
(4) Safe handling and disposal of sharps
(5) Waste and linen management
(6) Safe management of body fluid spills

These practices are the most fundamental and essential of all infection prevention precautions and should be applied consistently by all healthcare staff.

REFERENCES

Ayliffe, G.A.J., Babb, J.R. and Quoraishi, A.H. (1978) A test for hygienic hand disinfection. *Journal of Clinical Pathology*, **31**, 923.

Babb, J.R., Davis, J.G. and Ayliffe, G.A.J. (1983) Contamination of protective clothing and nurses' uniforms in an isolation ward. *Journal of Hospital Infection*, **4** (2), 149–157.

Blackmore, M.A. (1989) A comparison of hand drying methods. *Catering and Health*, **1**, 189–198.

Callaghan, I. (1998) Bacterial contamination of nurses' uniforms: a study. *Nursing Standard*, **13** (1), 37–42.

Department of Environment (1991) *Environmental Protection Act 1990, Section 34: Waste Management, the Duty of Care: Code of Practice.* HMSO, London.

Department of Health (1995) *HSG (95) 18: Hospital Laundry Arrangements for Used and Infected Linen.* Department of Health, Wetherby.

Department of Health (2005) *Guidance for Pandemic Influenza: Infection Control in Hospitals and Primary Care Settings* Available at: http://www.dh.gov.uk/assetRoot/04/12/17/54/04121754.pdf (accessed 22 November 2006).

Department of Health (2006) *Health Technical Memorandum 07–01: Safe Management of Healthcare Waste.* Available at: www.dh.gov.uk/en/Publicationsandstatistics/Publications/PublicationsPolicyAndGuidance/DH_063274 (accessed 1 April 2007).

Girou, E., Chai, S.H.T., Oppein, F. *et al.* (2004) Misuse of gloves: the foundation for poor compliance with hand hygiene and potential for microbial transmission. *Journal of Hospital Infection*, **57**, 162–169.

Gould, D. (1994) Making sense of hand hygiene. *The Journal of Infection Control Nursing – Nursing Times*, **90** (30), 63–64.

Health and Safety Executive (1999) *Control of Substances Hazardous to Health (COSHH) (Amendments) Act.* Health and Safety Executive, London.

Health and Safety Executive (1999) *Safe Disposal of Clinical Waste.* The Stationery Office, Norwich.

Health Protection Agency (2004) *Avian Influenza* Available at: http://www.hpa.org.uk/infections/topics_az/influenza/avian/ (accessed 22 November 2006).

Health Protection Scotland (2006a) *Hand Hygiene Policy and Procedure.* Available at: http://www.documents.hps.scot.nhs.uk/hai/infection-control/sicp/handhygiene/mic-p-handhygiene-2006-02.pdf (accessed 12 January 2007).

Health Protection Scotland (2006b) *Personal Protective Equipment Policy and Procedure.* Available at: http://www.documents.hps.scot.nhs.uk/hai/infection-control/sicp/ppe/mic-p-ppe-2006-02.pdf (accessed 12 January 2007).

Health Protection Scotland (2006c) *Occupational Exposure Management, Including Sharps Policy and Procedure.* Available at: http://www.documents.hps.scot.nhs.uk/hai/infection-control/sicp/occexposure/mic-p-occexposure-2006-02.pdf (accessed 12 January 2007).

Health Protection Scotland (2006d) *Safe Disposal of Waste: Policy and Procedure.* Available at: http://www.documents.hps.scot.nhs.uk/

hai/infection-control/sicp/waste/mic-p-waste-2006-02.pdf (accessed 12 January 2007).

Health Protection Scotland (2006e) *Safe Management of Linen Policy and Procedure*. Available at: http://www.documents.hps.scot.nhs.uk/ hai/infection-control/sicp/linen/mic-p-linen-2006-02.pdf (accessed 12 January 2007).

Infection Control Nurses Association (2002a) *Guidelines for Hand Hygiene*. Infection Control Nurses Association, Bathgate.

Infection Control Nurses Association (2002b) *Protective Clothing: Principles and Guidance*. Infection Control Nurses Association, Bathgate.

Infection Control Nurses Association (2003) *Reducing Sharps Injuries: Prevention and Risk Management*. Infection Control Nurses Association, Bathgate.

Infection Control Nurses Association (2004) *Audit Tools for Monitoring Infection Control Standards 2004*. Available at: www.icna.co.uk (accessed 26 November 2006).

Kownatzki, E. (2003) Hand hygiene and skin health. *Journal of Hospital Infection*, **55** (4), 239–245.

Larson, E. (1989) Hand washing: it's essential – even when you use gloves. *American Journal of Nursing*, **9**, 934–939.

Manian, F.A., Meyer, L. and Jenne, J. (1996) *Clostridium difficile* contamination of blood pressure cuffs: a call for a closer look at gloving practices in the era of universal precautions. *Infection Control Hospital Epidemiology*, **17** (3), 180–182.

McGuckin, M., Waterman, R., Storr, I.J. *et al.* (2001) Evaluation of a patient-empowering hand hygiene programme in the UK. *Journal of Hospital Infection*, **48** (3), 222–227.

Medical Devices Agency (1996) *Latex Sensitisation in the Healthcare Setting: Use of Latex Gloves (DB[960]))*. The Stationery Office, London.

National Audit Office (2003) *A Safer Place to Work: Improving the Management of Health and Safety Risks to Staff in NHS Trusts*. Available at: http://www.nao.org.uk/publications/nao_reports/02-03/ 0203623.pdf (accessed 23 November 2006).

Perry, C. and Gore, J. (1997) Now wash your hands please. *Nursing Times*, **93** (9), 64–68.

Perry, C., Marshall, R. and Jones, E. (2001) Bacterial contamination of uniforms. *Journal of Hospital Infection*, **38**, 238–241.

Pratt, R.J., Pellowe, C.M., Wilson, J.A., Loveday, H.P., Jones, S.R., McDougall, C. and Wilcox, M.H. (2007) epic2: national evidence based guidelines for preventing healthcare associated infections in NHS hospitals in England. *Journal of Hospital Infection*, **65** (Suppl. 1, Feb.), S1–64.

Public Health Laboratory Service (2002) Guidelines for public health management of meningococcal disease in the UK. *Communicable Disease and Public Health*, **5** (3), 187–204.

Rampling, A., Wiseman, S., Davis, L. *et al.* (2001) Evidence that hospital hygiene is important in the control of methicillin resistant *Staphylococcus aureus*. *Journal of Hospital Infection*, **49** (2), 109–116.

Royal College of Nursing (undated) *Uniforms: Infection Control Issues*. Available at: http://www.rcn.org.uk/resources/mrsa/healthcarestaff/uniforms/infectioncontrol.php (accessed 22 November 2006).

Statutory Instrument 588 (1992) *Controlled Waste Regulations*. HMSO, London.

Taylor, L. (1978) An evaluation of handwashing techniques 1. *Nursing Times*, 12 Jan., 54–55.

Telfer-Brunton, W.A. (1995) Infection and hospital laundry. *Lancet*, **345**, 1574–1575.

The Hazardous Waste (England and Wales) Regulations (2005) *Statutory Instrument 2005 No. 894*. The Stationery Office, London.

The Interdepartmental Working Group on Tuberculosis (1998) *The Prevention and Control of Tuberculosis in the United Kingdom: UK Guidance on the Prevention and Control of (1) HIV-related Tuberculosis and (2) Drug-resistant, including Multiple Drug-resistant, Tuberculosis*. Department of Health, London.

Truscott, W. (1995) They are not just gloves: a guideline on proper use. *Chicago Dental Society Review*, **88** (2), 22–29.

United Kingdom Health Departments (1998) *Guidance for Clinical Healthcare Workers: Protection Against Infection With Blood Borne Viruses*. The Stationery Office, London.

Weernink, A., Severin, W.P., Tjernberg, I. and Dijkshoorn, L. (1995) Pillows, an unexpected source of Acinetobacter. *Journal of Hospital Infection*, **29** (3), 189–199.

World Health Organization (2005) *WHO Guidelines on Hand Hygiene in Health Care (Advanced Draft): a Summary*. Available at: http://www.who.int/patientsafety/information_centre/ghhad_download/en/ (accessed on 1 April 2007).

6 | Specific and Common Infections

INTRODUCTION
Although the application of general infection prevention principles, as described in Chapter 5, will prevent many healthcare associated infections, there is a need to consider additional precautions for some specific infections. This chapter covers the most common and important of these infections that are likely to be encountered in hospital settings.

LEARNING OBJECTIVES
By the end of this chapter you will be able to describe patient care and infection prevention requirements related to:

❏ Meticillin resistant *Staphylococcus aureus*
❏ *Clostridium difficile*
❏ Tuberculosis
❏ Glycopeptide resistant enterococci
❏ Creutzfeldt-Jakob and variant CJD
❏ Meningococcal meningitis
❏ Multi-resistant Gram negative organisms including extended spectrum β-lactamase producing organisms (ESBL)
❏ Norovirus

METICILLIN RESISTANT *STAPHYLOCOCCUS AUREUS* (MRSA)
Staphylococcus aureus is a Gram positive aerobic bacterium that is spherical in shape. It is non-motile and does not form spores. In humans it can be found in up to 33% of the population and generally colonises the nose, perineum and non-intact skin of carriers. It can also be found in the environment in a hospital, particularly in areas where dust accumulates. Meticillin resistant *Staphylo-*

coccus aureus (MRSA) is a strain of *S. aureus* that is resistant to antibiotics which are usually used to treat infections caused by these bacteria, including flucloxacillin. MRSA was first identified in 1959, but did not cause many outbreaks of infection until the 1980s, when these outbreaks were largely confined to hospitals in the London area. In the early 1990s, levels of MRSA began to rise and outbreaks of epidemic strains of MRSA were seen in hospitals across the UK. Two particular strains of MRSA, EMRSA-15 and EMRSA-16 were identified as causing most increased cases of infection (Ayliffe *et al.*, 1998). From 1997 to 2005, 64% of all *S. aureus* wound infections were caused by MRSA (Health Protection Agency, 2006a). This rise in cases is of concern to hospitals as antibiotic therapy is limited, there are financial costs associated with treatment and management, and there is a great fear amongst patients and the public of acquiring this infection. Although cases of MRSA with mild resistance to vancomycin have been seen in the UK, there have been no cases of fully vancomycin resistant MRSA (VRSA) seen in the UK to date. Worldwide, cases of VRSA have been seen in Japan and the US (Coia *et al.*, 2006), making prevention and control of MRSA an even greater priority for hospitals.

MRSA is predominantly spread in the hospital setting by contact, with hands being the prime route of transmission. Contaminated equipment and airborne spread from skin scales and dust can lead to transmission of infection in hospitals. The types of infection caused by MRSA include:

- Wound infections
- Urinary tract infections
- Skin infections (impetigo and boils)
- Bloodstream infections (bacteraemia or septicaemia)
- Infections related to invasive devices (e.g. peripheral venous cannulae)
- Pneumonia

Prevention of MRSA infection is achieved by applying the standard infection prevention practices described in Chapter 5. In addition, the following additional practices may be applied (Coia *et al.*, 2006).

Patient placement

Patient placement is dependent on the location of the patient in hospital and based on the risk to other patients in the ward/department.

High risk areas include:

- Intensive care units
- Neonatal intensive care units
- Burn units
- Transplantation units
- Cardiothoracic units
- Orthopaedic and trauma units
- Vascular surgery units
- Renal units
- Regional, national and international referral units

Patients must be isolated in a single room wherever possible. Single rooms with en suite facilities are also preferable. It may be possible to cohort patients together in a designated area of a unit if there is more than one MRSA positive patient. The door should be kept closed wherever possible and must always be closed during activities that may generate dust and aerosols, such as bedmaking or wound dressings.

Medium risk areas include:

- Surgical wards
- Admission wards
- Paediatric wards
- Medical wards

Patients should be isolated in a single room, with the door kept closed, if possible. Single rooms with en suite facilities are also preferable. It may be possible to cohort patients together in a designated area of a unit if there is more than one MRSA positive patient. The door should be kept closed wherever possible and must always be closed during activities that may generate dust and aerosols, such as bedmaking or wound dressings.

Low risk areas include:

- Psychiatric areas
- Psychogeriatric areas
- Long-term care facilities

Patient placement in a single room may not be necessary in these areas. This will depend on the level of risk to other patients; for example if patients have wounds or indwelling catheters single room isolation would be preferable.

Discontinuation of isolation

Patients should be considered infected or colonised with MRSA until three consecutive sets of screening swabs, taken when treatment has ceased, have tested negative.

Staff

There is no restriction on staff. It is sensible to avoid having staff who have skin conditions such as eczema or psoriasis from caring for MRSA positive patients due to the increased risk of them becoming colonised.

Visiting staff, for example physiotherapists, should be given instructions on precautions that are required before they enter the room.

Screening

Admission screening should be considered for the following groups of patients (DoH, 2006):

- All patients admitted to an intensive care unit – on admission and weekly if their stay is prolonged
- All patients undergoing elective orthopaedic surgery
- All patients undergoing elective cardiothoracic surgery
- All patients undergoing vascular surgery
- All patients on renal dialysis – before starting dialysis and on a regular basis (agreed locally) whilst dialysis is ongoing
- Patients from nursing and residential care facilities
- Patients with chronic conditions that require frequent hospital re-admissions

Screening specimens should be obtained from:

- Nose
- Skin lesions, wounds and insertion sites of invasive devices
- Groin/perineum
- Catheter urine
- Sputum if the patient has a productive cough

Post-treatment screening

This should be carried out once the patient has completed a course of treatment if testing for clearance of MRSA is required. Samples should be taken from the sites detailed above at weekly intervals. Three consecutive negative samples are required before a patient can be declared free of MRSA. However, it is still possible for patients who have been declared negative for MRSA to subsequently be MRSA positive again, either through recolonisation or through sampling failing to detect very low levels of MRSA.

Treatment

Patients with infections will be treated systemically with appropriate antibiotics. Patients who are colonised and infected generally require topical decolonisation therapy as follows:

Nasal decolonisation Mupirocin 2% is applied to each nostril three times daily for five days. If applied correctly, patients should be able to taste mupirocin at the back of the throat. Mupirocin should not be given for longer than prescribed due to the risk of resistance developing.

Throat decolonisation Treatment should be given on the advice of a microbiologist and will often consist of antibiotic therapy.

Skin decolonisation Treatment is daily bathing, washing or showering in an antiseptic:

- 4% chlorhexidine body wash
- 7.5% povidone iodine
- 2% triclosan

This should be applied neat to moistened skin daily for five days. Patients with skin conditions may require other treatments that will be prescribed on the advice of a dermatologist.

Patients' bedding, clothing and towels should be changed at the end of a course of treatment.

Protective clothing

- Gloves should be worn where there is a risk of contact with bodily fluids and for handling of contaminated linen or dressings.
- Aprons should be worn by all staff who will be handling the patient or who will have contact with their immediate environment, for example cleaning staff.
- Masks are generally not required, but may occasionally be needed for procedures that are likely to generate aerosols, for example chest physiotherapy.

Hand hygiene

Hands should be decontaminated by either hand washing or the use of an alcohol gel before and after contact with the patient or their immediate environment.

Cleaning procedures

General cleaning

A good standard of general cleaning on a daily basis is required to keep levels of dust at a minimum. Detergent and water is generally sufficient, but disinfectants may be used in accordance with local policy.

Discharge cleaning

The room should undergo a thorough and enhanced clean to include areas where dust may collect, including radiators and ventilator ducts. Detergent and water is generally sufficient, but disinfectants may be used in accordance with local policy. Curtains should be removed and laundered.

It may be useful to use a discharge cleaning checklist (Figure 6.1) to ensure the room is adequately cleaned.

RECORD OF TERMINAL CLEANING OF ROOM/BEDSPACE AFTER TRANSFER/DISCHARGE OF A PATIENT			
Patient: Moved from:		**Bedspace/Side room:**	
NURSING TASK	**NURSE SIG.**	**DOMESTIC TASK**	**DOM. SIG.**
Wear gloves and apron.		Wear gloves and apron.	
Remove all patient's property and pack/dispose of property.		Remove bed space/room curtains and treat as infective (red alginate bag in red plastic linen bag).	
Remove bed linen and treat as infective (red alginate bag in red plastic linen bag).		Ensure that nursing duties have been carried out before cleaning.	
Dispose of all single use equipment: O2 tubing/liners. Wash down oxygen and suction units with Actichlor Plus and dry thoroughly with blue roll.		Wash all surfaces with Actichlor Plus – see poster for correct dilution. Use disposable cloths and rinse regularly between surfaces.	
Wash down all equipment and furniture with Actichlor Plus, rinsing cloth regularly. *Do not* soak equipment. Follow manufacturers' instructions for dilution of Actichlor Plus. Wipe over all surfaces and equipment and allow to air dry or dry with blue roll.		Paper towels and hand washing agents *do not* need to be removed from holders. Soap holders and alcohol hand rub dispensers should be wiped over.	
Any equipment suitable for sterilisation should be sent back to sterile services in a designated bag/container.		Ensure that all surfaces are completely clean and dry. Clean floor with Actichlor Plus and leave to dry.	

Figure 6.1 Discharge cleaning checklist.

Check pillows and mattress. Ensure that pressure relieving mattress is cleaned with Actichlor Plus (check with rental company that mattress can tolerate Actichlor Plus) before it is returned to rental company for decontamination. Check that pillow covers and ordinary mattresses are intact and clean with Actichlor Plus and dry. Arrange for domestic to clean the bedspace/room.		Clean bedframe with Actichlor Plus and dry. Remove gloves and disposable apron after cleaning the room and *wash hands* with soap and water Dispose of cleaning cloths. Ensure mop heads are laundered before reuse. Clean all other cleaning equipment, e.g. buckets thoroughly. Replace curtains with a clean set.	
After cleaning, the nurse in charge must inspect the room/bedspace		Inform nursing staff that the room/bedspace has been cleaned	
WASH HANDS WITH SOAP and WATER		**WASH HANDS WITH SOAP and WATER**	

Figure 6.1 *Continued*

Equipment

Where possible, equipment should be single use or dedicated for the individual patient's use. Reusable equipment must be adequately decontaminated before using on another patient (refer to Chapter 16).

Crockery and cutlery may be washed in the dishwasher in the usual manner.

Waste

All waste should be discarded as clinical waste.

Linen

Great care should be taken in handling linen to prevent shedding of dust and skin scales. All linen should be treated as infected.

Transfers to other wards and departments

Patients with MRSA should not be transferred to other wards until it is clinically necessary.

Visits to other departments, such as radiology, should be kept to a minimum. Where visits are necessary the receiving department must be told in advance and the following principles applied:

- Skin lesions should be covered with an occlusive dressing.
- Transporting staff, for example porters, should wear disposable aprons only when they are in contact with the patient; these should be discarded immediately contact has ceased.
- Transporting staff do not need to wear gloves unless they have obvious lesions on their hands.
- Hand hygiene by hand washing or alcohol gel is necessary after patient and equipment contact.
- Trolleys or wheelchairs used for patient transfers should be decontaminated before use on another patient.
- Patients should not wait in holding areas with other patients, wherever possible, but should be brought to the department immediately before and returned to their isolation room immediately after treatments or investigations.

Visitors

There is no restriction on visitors. Protective clothing (gloves and aprons) need only be worn when carrying out bodily care activities. All visitors should be instructed on the precautions required, including hand hygiene on leaving the room.

Discharge

MRSA should not delay a patient's discharge if they are medically fit. The GP and/or district nurse should be informed of the patient's MRSA status. The following information will be required:

- Date and site of initial MRSA positive specimen (if during this admission)
- Details of any actual infection
- Date and results of most recent MRSA screen

- Any treatment that needs to continue, including starting date, dose and stop date
- Details of any follow-up screening required

MRSA treatments may not need to be continued after discharge. Advice should be sought from the local infection control team.

Patients and carers should be advised that there are no specific restrictions or precautions needed for patients being discharged to their own home. Patients should be advised that if they require further hospitalisation or healthcare treatments that they should inform staff prior to treatment wherever possible.

Ambulance staff should be informed in advance. There is generally no restriction on ambulance transport; however, MRSA positive patients should not be transported with other patients who may be more susceptible, such as renal patients.

Deceased patients
No specific precautions are required.

CLOSTRIDIUM DIFFICILE
Clostridum difficile is a Gram positive anaerobic rod shaped bacterium. It is non-motile but it is spore forming, enhancing its ability to survive in a hospital environment. It colonises the gut and can be found in 2% of the healthy adult population (Wilcox, 2003). This rate of colonisation increases to 10–20% of elderly people, particularly if they have had contact with healthcare facilities. *C. difficile* can be found colonising the gut of younger children but is rarely associated with actual disease. Environmental contamination is common with *C. difficile* and the bacteria have been found in soil, swimming pool and tap water, on nurses' uniforms, blood pressure monitoring cuffs, thermometers and on commodes (Manian *et al.*, 1996; Barnett *et al.*, 1999). Spores are able to survive in the environment for many months and can reactivate in the right conditions to cause cases of infection. Levels of *C. difficile* have been rising in the UK, with 49 850 reported cases in England and Wales and Northern Ireland in 2005 (Health Protection Agency, 2006b). This increase is of concern to hospitals as *C. difficile* infection increases a patient's stay in hospital by on

average 21 days, and is particularly debilitating to the elderly (Wilcox, 2003). More recently, strains of *C. difficile* (type 027) have been found in UK hospitals that appear to cause more severe disease and have led to outbreaks of infection (Das and Jumaa, 2006). These strains may be less susceptible to treatments, causing frequent relapses in affected patients.

Transmission is by contact and the faecal-oral route. Infection manifests itself in patients in a range of severity:

- Diarrhoea – mild to severe
- Pseudomembranous colitis
- Toxic megacolon

Infection can be severe enough in some cases for patients to require a colectomy or for bowel perforation to occur.

Prevention of *C. difficile* is through adoption of standard infection control principles and strict control of antibiotic therapy in hospitals. Certain groups of antibiotics are implicated in *C. difficile* infection more than others. These include:

- Cephalosporins
- Clindamycin
- Ampicillin
- Amoxycillin
- Co-trimoxazole
- Macrolides
- Tetracyclines
- Fluoroquinolones

Patients who are *C. difficile* positive, but do not have diarrhoea, do not require specific precautions. For patients with diarrhoea, the following additional precautions may be applied (Department of Health and Public Health Laboratory Service, 1994).

Patient placement

Isolation in a single room is strongly recommended. Where possible this should be with en suite facilities. The door need not be kept closed all the time but should be closed during toileting and hygiene activities as well as bedmaking.

Discontinuation of isolation

Isolation may be discontinued when patients have been free of diarrhoea or have returned to their normal bowel habit for 72 hours or with the agreement of the infection control team if a patient's diarrhoea appears to be lessening. Follow-up samples are not used to determine when isolation can cease as patients may continue to excrete the bacteria for some months; however, the risk of cross infection is minimal if the patient does not have active diarrhoea.

Staff

There is no general restriction on staff; however, it is sensible to avoid having staff that are currently taking a course of antibiotics from caring for positive patients.

Visiting staff, for example physiotherapists, should be given instructions on precautions that are required before they enter the room.

Treatment

Any antibiotics that the patient is currently receiving should be stopped wherever possible.

Treatment is generally a course of metronidazole or vancomycin given orally. Intravenous metronidazole is occasionally used but vancomycin will not be effective against *C. difficile* if given intravenously.

Patients with severe *C. difficile* disease may be prescribed albumin, immunoglobulins or steroids.

Protective clothing

- Gloves should be worn for all direct contact with the patient, equipment and the immediate environment.
- Plastic aprons should be worn for all direct patient contact, as well as for contact with equipment and the immediate environment.
- Masks and eye protection need only be worn in accordance with risk assessment for standard precautions.

Hand Hygiene

Hands of all personnel entering and leaving the room should be decontaminated by hand washing under running water. An antiseptic hand wash solution should be used out of preference. Alcohol hand rubs should not be used as they have limited effectiveness against *C. difficile* spores.

Patients must be encouraged to wash their hands after using the toilet and before eating to reduce the risk of re-infection.

Cleaning procedures

General cleaning

A good standard of general cleaning on a daily basis is required to keep levels of spores at a minimum. A disinfectant, for example chlorine, should be used for general cleaning.

Discharge cleaning

The room should undergo a thorough and enhanced clean. *C. difficile* spores have been found to survive in a ward environment for five months (Fekety *et al.*, 1981). Therefore, it is vital that an adequate discharge clean is performed; a discharge checklist may be useful. A disinfectant, for example chlorine, should be used. Curtains should be removed and laundered.

Equipment

Where possible, equipment should be single use or dedicated for the individual patient's use; in particular, a commode should be dedicated for individual use. Reusable equipment must be adequately decontaminated before being used on another patient (refer to Chapter 16). Particular care should be taken to ensure sanitary equipment is adequately decontaminated before further use.

Crockery and cutlery may be washed in the dishwasher in the usual manner.

Waste

All waste should be discarded as clinical waste.

Linen

All linen should be treated as infected. Patients' soiled clothing should not be laundered locally. If soiled clothing is to be taken home for laundering this should be placed in a plastic bag and relatives advised to launder it at the maximum wash code the item will allow and separate from other laundry.

Transfers to other wards and departments

Patients with *C. difficile* diarrhoea should not be transferred to other wards unless it is clinically necessary.

Visits to other departments, such as radiology, should be kept to a minimum. Where visits are necessary the receiving department must be told in advance and the following principles applied:

• Transporting staff, for example porters, should wear disposable gloves and aprons only when they are in contact with the patient; these should be discarded immediately contact has ceased.
• Hand hygiene by hand washing is necessary after patient and equipment contact.
• Trolleys or wheelchairs used for patient transfers should be decontaminated before use on another patient.
• Patients should not wait in holding areas with other patients, wherever possible, but should be brought to the department immediately before and returned to their isolation room immediately after treatments or investigations.

Visitors

There is no general restriction on visitors. It may be prudent to advise against visiting if visitors are currently receiving a course of antibiotics. Protective clothing (gloves and aprons) need only be worn when carrying out bodily care activities. All visitors should be instructed on the precautions required, including hand washing on leaving the room.

Discharge

Patients with *C. difficile* can be discharged when they are medically fit. The GP and/or district nurse should be informed. They should be advised that if the patient develops diarrhoea in the future, particularly in relation to receiving antibiotics, that *C. difficile* should be considered and the appropriate advice sought.

Patients and carers should be advised that there are no specific restrictions or precautions needed for patients being discharged to their own home. Ambulance staff should be informed in advance; there is generally no restriction on ambulance transport.

Deceased patients

No specific precautions are required.

TUBERCULOSIS

Tuberculosis (TB) is caused by the bacterium *Mycobacterium tuberculosis*. This is a straight or slightly curved rod that is non-motile and non-spore forming. The outer layer of the bacterial cell is waxy and cannot be stained using the standard Gram staining in the laboratory. Instead, it is identified using an alcohol acid fast stain. Laboratory staining reports for *M. tuberculosis* and other mycobacteria can also refer to this as Ziehl Nielsen (ZN) stain.

TB is predominantly a pulmonary disease, but infection can be found in other areas of the body, including lymph nodes, kidney, bladder and joints. Infection is more common in ethnic groups from high prevalence countries, including sub-Saharan Africa and the Indian subcontinent, the homeless population and people from low socio-economic background; it is also associated with human immunodeficiency virus (HIV). Control measures in the UK in the nineteenth century led to a decline in cases of TB. Although overall cases of TB have risen again in the UK, this is largely due to infections acquired outside the UK (DoH, 2004).

TB is spread by the airborne route in droplet form. Cases of TB transmission in hospitals have been reported, associated with the carrying out of aerosol generating procedures on open wards caring for HIV positive patients (Kent *et al.*, 1994). Healthcare staff have been reported as acquiring infection from TB positive patients during their work (Bolyard *et al.*, 1998). More recently, strains of antibiotic resistant TB have been recognised. Multi-drug resistant TB (MDR-TB) is where the bacteria are resistant to two or more of the drugs usually used for TB treatment, generally isoniazid or rifampicin with or without other drugs (The Interdepartmental Working Group on Tuberculosis, 1998).

Primary infection from TB occurs as a lesion in the lung within 4–12 weeks after exposure to the bacterium. This primary infection may progress to pulmonary TB or infection at other sites within two years of infection. The primary infection can lie dormant for many years and can then reactivate to cause latent infection. Signs and symptoms of pulmonary TB include:

- Productive cough
- General malaise
- Weight loss
- Night sweats
- Bloodstained sputum
- Chest pain

Infection is diagnosed either by the examination of sputum or other body fluid/tissue, or from chest radiography. TB disease is classified as either:

- **Open/infectious** – the presence of TB bacteria in the sputum, identified by ZN or alcohol acid fast stain, with symptoms of a productive cough

- **Closed/non-infectious** – the presence of TB bacteria in other body fluids or tissue, identified by ZN or alcohol acid fast stain, or the presence of TB bacteria in sputum identified by culture (growing the TB bacteria in the laboratory)

Infection control procedures will differ depending on whether a patient has open or closed TB and the risk of infection to other patients in the ward/department.

Prevention of transmission of TB is through prompt recognition of patients who could have open TB and then taking the appropriate isolation precautions. In the UK it is also recommended that healthcare workers are offered BCG vaccination on commencing employment. The following additional infection control measures may be applied to prevent spread of TB in hospitals (The Interdepartmental Working Group on Tuberculosis, 1996, 1998; Joint Tuberculosis Committee of the British Thoracic Society, 2000; Royal College of Physicians, 2006).

Patient placement

Patient placement is dependent on whether the patient has open or closed TB and whether it is thought to be drug resistant (see Table 6.1).

The door should be kept closed and the patient should not leave the room unless clinically necessary.

A negative pressure room is specifically designed and maintained so that the air pressure outside the room is higher than the air pressure in the room. When the door is opened the difference in pressure means that air from outside the room is drawn in so that there is no risk of droplets of TB releasing from the room. Air is extracted from the room either through a filter or is discharged from a location where there is no risk of other patients coming into contact with the air extract.

Table 6.1 Isolation for TB positive patients.

	Immunocompetent patients on ward			Immunocompromised patients on ward		
	Infectious	Potentially infectious	Non-infectious	Infectious	Potentially infectious	Non-infectious
Drug sensitive	Single room	Open ward	Open ward	Negative pressure room	Open ward	Single room
Drug resistant	Single room	Open ward	Open ward	Negative pressure room	Single room	Open ward
Multi-drug resistant (MDR-TB)	Negative pressure room	Single room	Open ward	Negative pressure room	Negative pressure room	Single room

Discontinuation of isolation

Non-resistant TB   Isolation can usually be discontinued when the patient has received 14 days of appropriate drug treatment.

MDR-TB   Isolation should be continued until three consecutive sputum specimens have tested negative for the TB bacteria by the ZN or acid fast stain and with the approval of the infection control and respiratory teams.

Staff
Only staff that have received BCG vaccination should care for patients with open TB. This applies to visiting staff, for example occupational therapists.

Treatment
Treatment is by a combination of the following drugs:

- Rifampicin
- Pyrazinamide
- Isoniazid
- Streptomycin
- Ethambutol
- Ethionamide
- Prothionamide

They are taken in combination to reduce the risk of resistance, which is high with TB. Courses of treatment can last up to six months.

Protective clothing

- Gloves should be worn for handling of the patient and their immediate environment and for contact with secretions, contaminated dressings and linen.
- Aprons should be worn by all staff who will be handling the patient or who will have contact with their immediate environment, for example cleaning staff.
- Masks/respirators are required for:

— Cough-inducing or aerosol generating procedures
— Physiotherapy
— Prolonged care of patients who are unable to control their cough

A high-level filtration mask (FFP2 minimum and FFP3 for known or strongly suspected MDR-TB) should be worn (see Chapter 5).

Hand hygiene

Hands should be decontaminated by either hand washing or the use of an alcohol gel before and after contact with the patient or their immediate environment.

Cleaning procedures

General cleaning
A good standard of general cleaning on a daily basis is required. Detergent and water is generally sufficient, but disinfectants may be used in accordance with local policy.

Discharge cleaning
The room should undergo a thorough and enhanced clean. Detergent and water is generally sufficient but disinfectants may be used in accordance with local policy. Curtains should be removed and laundered.

Equipment

Where possible, equipment should be single use or dedicated for the individual patient's use. Reusable equipment must be adequately decontaminated before using on another patient (refer to Chapter 16).

Crockery and cutlery may be washed in the dishwasher in the usual manner.

Waste

All waste should be discarded as clinical waste.

Linen

All linen should be treated as infected.

Transfers to other wards and departments

Patients with open TB should not be transferred to other wards until it is clinically necessary.

Visits to other departments, such as radiology, should be kept to a minimum. Where visits are necessary the receiving department must be told in advance and the following principles applied:

- The patient should wear a surgical mask if they are unable to control their cough or cannot be relied upon to cough into a tissue.
- Transporting staff, for example porters, should wear disposable gloves and aprons only when they are in contact with the patient; these should be discarded immediately contact has ceased.
- Hand hygiene by hand washing or alcohol gel is necessary after patient and equipment contact.
- Trolleys or wheelchairs used for patient transfers should be decontaminated before use on another patient.
- Patients must not wait in holding areas with other patients, they should be brought to the department immediately before and returned to their isolation room immediately after treatments or investigations.

Visitors

Visitors should be restricted to those who have had close contact with the patient before diagnosis.

All close contacts of the patient will be followed up by a communicable disease control team to ensure they are not also infectious or incubating TB.

Protective clothing (gloves and aprons) need only be worn when carrying out bodily care activities. All visitors should be instructed on the precautions required, including hand hygiene on leaving the room.

Specimens

All specimens sent to the laboratory should be identified to the laboratory as a biohazard, either through the use of a biohazard sticker, a tick-box on the request form, or both.

Discharge

If a patient with open TB is being discharged before they have completed 14 days of treatment then the local communicable disease control team should be notified; they will advise on any precautions that may be necessary.

Ambulance staff should be informed in advance if the patient is known to still have open TB.

Deceased patients

It is advisable that a body bag is used and the mortuary staff informed of the patient's infectious status.

GLYCOPEPTIDE RESISTANT ENTEROCOCCI

Enterococci are Gram positive aerobic bacteria. They are non-spore forming and are generally non-motile. Vancomycin is a glycopeptide antibiotic; the terms vancomycin (VRE) and glyco-peptide resistant enterococci (GRE) are used interchangeably when referring to these bacteria. GRE were first identified in 1998. *Enterococcus faecalis and Enterococcus faecium* are the types of this bacteria that are most commonly associated with infection in hospitalised patients. *E. faecalis and E. faecium* can be found in the gut of normal healthy individuals. Although the resistant strains of these bacteria are no more likely to cause infection than non-resistant strains, the fact that they are antibiotic resistant makes them more difficult to treat. GRE infections are more commonly found in wards and departments where vancomycin is frequently used, for example in renal units.

Infections caused by GRE are often endogenous, that is caused by the patient's own bacteria. Cross infection can occur in hospitals by contact spread, on the hands of healthcare workers, or on inadequately decontaminated equipment. The following infections can be caused by GRE:

- Wound infections
- Urinary tract infections
- Septicaemia

Asymptomatic carriage of GRE is common (Murray, 1990) and patients can continue to excrete GRE in faeces. Eradication of

GRE carriage has not been found to be effective. Therefore, it is not possible to give decolonisation therapy, as with MRSA.

Limiting the use of glycopeptide antibiotics, in particular vancomycin, is important in prevention of infection. In addition to standard precautions, the following additional precautions are often applied (Centers for Disease Prevention and Control, 1995; Cookson *et al.*, 2006).

Patient placement

Patient placement is dependent on a risk assessment of whether the patient has diarrhoea or evidence of infection (Figure 6.2) and

Patient isolation algorithm

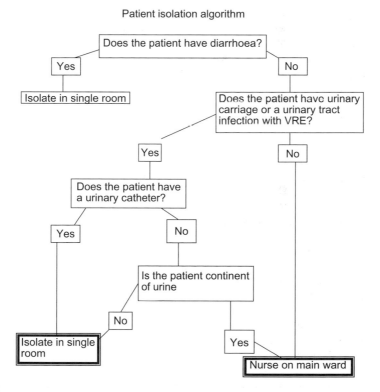

Figure 6.2 Algorithm for isolation of GRE positive patient.

the location of the patient in hospital. Where single room isolation is used, the door need not be kept closed all the time, but should be closed for dust and aerosol generating activities, such as bed-making and physiotherapy.

Discontinuation of isolation

Testing for clearance of GRE may be helpful in determining when isolation can be discontinued. Specimens of stool, urine and swabs from broken areas of skin may be requested. As discontinuation of isolation depends on a variety of factors, advice should be sought from the infection control team.

Staff

There is no restriction on staff.

Visiting staff, for example physiotherapists, should be given instructions on precautions that are required before they enter the room.

Treatment

Patients with infections will be treated systemically with appropriate antibiotics.

Protective clothing

- Gloves should be worn for all contact with the patient and their immediate environment.
- Aprons should be worn by all staff who will be handling the patient or who will have contact with their immediate environment, for example cleaning staff.
- Masks are generally not required but should be worn when a risk assessment under standard precautions dictates.

Hand hygiene

Hands should be decontaminated by either hand washing or the use of an alcohol gel before and after contact with the patient or their immediate environment.

Cleaning procedures

General cleaning
A good standard of general cleaning on a daily basis is required to keep levels of environmental contamination at a minimum. A disinfectant, for example hypochlorite, should be used.

Discharge cleaning
The room should undergo a thorough and enhanced clean to include areas where dust may collect, including radiators and ventilator ducts. A disinfectant, for example hypochlorite, should be used. Curtains should be removed and laundered.

Equipment
Where possible equipment should be single use or dedicated for the individual patient's use. Reusable equipment must be adequately decontaminated before using on another patient (refer to Chapter 16). Enterococci have been found to be resistant to chemical disinfection (Bradley and Fraise, 1996); a heat process should be used wherever possible. This is particularly important for sanitary items such as bedpans and urine collection jugs.

Crockery and cutlery may be washed in the dishwasher in the usual manner.

Waste
All waste should be discarded as clinical waste.

Linen
All linen should be treated as infected.

Transfers to other wards and departments
Patients should not be transferred to other wards until it is clinically necessary.

Visits to other departments, such as radiology, should be kept to a minimum. Where visits are necessary the receiving department must be told in advance and the following principles applied:

- Transporting staff, for example porters, should wear disposable gloves and aprons only when they are in contact with the patient; these should be discarded immediately contact has ceased.
- Hand hygiene by hand washing or alcohol gel is necessary after patient and equipment contact.
- Trolleys or wheelchairs used for patient transfers should be decontaminated before use on another patient.
- Patients should not wait in holding areas with other patients, wherever possible, but should be brought to the department immediately before and returned to their isolation room immediately after treatments or investigations.

Visitors

There is no restriction on visitors. Protective clothing (gloves and aprons) need only be worn when carrying out bodily care activities. All visitors should be instructed on the precautions required, including hand hygiene on leaving the room.

Discharge

GRE should not delay a patient's discharge if they are medically fit. The GP and/or district nurse should be informed of the patient's GRE status. The following information will be required:

- Date and site of initial GRE positive specimen (if during this admission)
- Details of any actual infection
- Date and results of most recent GRE screen, if applicable

Patients and carers should be advised that there are no specific restrictions or precautions needed for patients being discharged to their own home. Patients should be advised that if they require further hospitalisation or healthcare treatments then they should inform staff prior to treatment wherever possible that they have been GRE positive.

Ambulance staff should be informed in advance. There is generally no restriction on ambulance transport; however, GRE positive patients should not be transported with other patients who may be more susceptible, such as renal patients.

Deceased patients
No specific precautions are required.

CREUTZFELDT-JAKOB DISEASE
Creutzfeldt-Jakob disease (CJD) is one of a group of diseases
known as transmissible spongiform encephalopathies (TSEs).
These are fatal degenerative brain diseases that are found in both
humans and animals. They are characterised by microscopic
holes in the grey matter of the brain, and in laboratory settings
have been found to be transmissible by mouth and by percutaneous inoculation.

The following TSEs have been identified in humans:

* Creutzfeldt-Jakob disease

   — Classical – occurs sporadically, no known cause
   — Familial – genetically linked
   — Iatrogenic – acquired through a healthcare procedure, for
     examples administration of contaminated human growth
     factor
   — Variant – linked to bovine spongiform encephalopathy
     (mad cow disease)

* Gerstmann Straussler-Scheinker syndrome
* Fatal familial insomnia
* Kuru – this is linked to ritualistic cannibalism

TSEs appear to be caused by unconventional infectious agents:
prion proteins. These do not have the same characteristics as
bacteria or viruses, but are proteins with abnormal folding. They
do not reproduce conventionally, but have the ability to alter the
protein in adjacent cells to become the same rogue protein as
prion. Prion proteins are resistant to the normal chemical and
physical methods used for disinfection and sterilisation. Therefore, specific precautions are necessary for patients undergoing
some invasive and surgical procedures.

Variant CJD (vCJD) is linked to bovine spongiform encephalopathy (mad cow disease) and primarily affects younger patients
than the sporadic form of CJD. Variant CJD often presents with

mood and psychiatric disturbances and with the following signs and symptoms:

- Alteration of sensation
- Disturbance of balance and movement
- Loss of memory and poor cognitive skills
- Communication problems
- Swallowing difficulties
- Visual and perceptual disturbances
- Seizures

A presumptive diagnosis can be made through blood tests, electroencephalographs, brain scans, neuro-imaging, psychometric tests and examination of cerebrospinal fluid. Final diagnosis can only currently be made through brain biopsy or post-mortem examination.

Table 6.2 details the number of deaths from CJD and vCJD to the end of 2005. CJD and vCJD are not transmitted through normal social and clinical contact. Transmission has occurred accidentally through human growth hormone, corneal transplants and the use of human dura mater grafts. The extent to which human tissues are infectious varies with CJD and vCJD (see Table 6.3).

Table 6.2 Deaths due to CJD and vCJD in the United Kingdom to end of 2005 (Source: www.dh.gov.uk).

Year	Deaths due to definite and probable CJD	Deaths due to definite and possible vCJD
2005	66	5
2004	58	9
2003	88	18
2002	77	17
2001	67	20
2000	54	28
1999	70	15
1998	71	18
1997	71	10
1996	50	10

Table 6.3 Level of infectivity and risk of transmission of CJD and vCJD in human tissues.

Level of infectivity	CJD	vCJD
High	• Brain • Spinal cord • Posterior eye	• Brain • Spinal cord • Posterior eye
Medium	• Anterior eye • Olfactory epithelium	• Anterior eye • Olfactory epithelium • Lymphoid tissue
Low	• All other tissues	• All other tissues

Standard precautions apply to the care of patients who are symptomatic with CJD and vCJD or who are either suspected of having a TSE or are at risk of a TSE. Additional precautions are required for surgical and invasive instrument use according to whether patients actually have the disease or are at risk of disease. Definitions for at risk, symptomatic and asymptomatic are given in Table 6.4.

The following additional precautions apply to CJD and vCJD patients in wards (Advisory Committee on Dangerous Pathogens and the Spongiform Encephalopathy Advisory Committee, 2003).

Patient placement
Isolation is not necessary.

Staff
No staff restrictions are necessary.

Protective clothing
This should follow standard precautions.

Hand hygiene
In accordance with standard precautions using either hand washing or alcohol hand gel.

Table 6.4 Definitions of CJD and vCJD for infection control purposes.

Symptomatic patients

- Those who fulfil the diagnostic criteria for definite, probable or possible CJD or vCJD
- Those who have symptoms of neurological disease where CJD or vCJD is being actively considered as a diagnosis.

Asymptomatic patients at risk from familial forms of CJD

- Those who have had one or more blood relatives affected by CJD or other TSE
- Those who have a relative known to have a genetic mutation indicative of familial CJD
- Those who have been shown by genetic testing to be at risk of developing CJD or other TSE

Asymptomatic patients potentially at risk from iatrogenic exposures

- Those who have received growth hormome derived from human pituitary glands
- Those who have received a graft of human dura mater
- Those who have been contacted through the CJD panel and been advised that they are at risk due to exposure to instruments used on blood, organs or tissues donated by a patient who developed CJD or vCJD

Specimens

Specimens taken using invasive procedures, for example blood sampling, should be carried out by experienced personnel.

All specimens sent to the laboratory should be identified to the laboratory as a biohazard, either through the use of a biohazard sticker, a tick-box on the request form or both.

Cleaning procedures

No specific precautions are required for general or discharge cleaning.

Spills of high risk body fluids, for example cerebrospinal fluid, should be decontaminated using either sodium hypochlorite containing 20000 ppm available chlorine or 1 M sodium hydroxide, with repeated wetting to the spillage area over one hour. All equipment used in clearing the spill should be incinerated.

Table 6.5 Decontamination procedures for invasive equipment used on CJD and vCJD patients.

Tissue infectivity	Status of patient			
CJD	**Definite/probable**	**Possible**	**At risk genetic**	**At risk iatrogenic**
High	Incinerate	Quarantine	Incinerate	Incinerate
Medium	Incinerate	Quarantine	Incinerate	Incinerate
Low	No special precautions	No special precautions	No special precautions	No special precautions
vCJD	**Definite/probable**	**Possible**		**At risk iatrogenic**
High	Incinerate	Quarantine		Incinerate
Medium	Incinerate	Quarantine		Incinerate
Low	No special precautions	No special precautions		No special precautions

Equipment

There are no specific requirements for general equipment.

Disposable equipment must be used for lumbar punctures. For other invasive procedures, disposable equipment should be used wherever possible. If reusable invasive equipment is used follow the procedures in Table 6.5.

Waste

There are no special precautions.

Linen

There are no special precautions.

Transfers to other wards and departments

There are no special precautions.

Visitors

No special precautions are necessary.

Discharge

If the diagnosis has been made during the current admission, the GP and district nurse should be informed. Guidance on management of CJD and vCJD in the community is available (DoH, undated).

Deceased patient

The mortuary should be informed, as post-mortems should only be carried out in a specialised mortuary.

Last offices should be performed as usual and the use of a body bag is not required.

MENINGOCOCCAL MENINGITIS

Meningococcal meningitis and septicaemia is caused by the bacterium *Neisseria meningitidis*. It is a Gram negative, aerobic bacterium that is non-spore forming and is motile through the use of flagellae. The bacteria can be found colonising the nasopharynx of 10% of the general population, but this may be up to 25% in young adults.

Transmission of the bacterium is by contact with droplets from the upper respiratory tract. The incubation period is 2–10 days, but disease progression can be rapid. Symptoms and signs of disease include:

- Malaise
- Pyrexia
- Vomiting
- Headache
- Photophobia
- Drowsiness
- Petechial rash that does not blanch under pressure

Transmission of meningococcal meningitis to other patients in a hospital setting has not been reported and the risk to healthcare workers is minimal. However, the following precautions should be applied (Public Health Laboratory Service, 2002).

Patient placement

Ideally, the patient should be nursed in a single room. This should be continued until they have received 48 hours of appropriate antibiotic therapy.

Staff

No restrictions on staff are necessary.

Visiting staff, for example physiotherapists, should be advised of the correct precautions to take.

Staff will only be considered for antibiotic prophylaxis if they have been in direct contact with the patient's respiratory secretions without having worn the appropriate protective clothing, for example emergency intubation without having worn a mask.

Treatment

Early treatment is highly recommended. If the GP has not already given benzyl penicillin, or chloramphenicol if they are allergic to this, then this should be given immediately.

Protective clothing

Gloves and aprons should be worn as per standard precautions.

Healthcare workers carrying out airway management, for example intubation or suctioning, should wear a fluid repellent theatre-type mask.

Hand hygiene

This should be before and after all patient contact, with either hand washing or the use of alcohol hand gel.

Cleaning procedures

These should be as per standard procedures.

Equipment

Closed system suction should be used to reduce the risk of staff being in contact with respiratory secretions.

Reusable equipment can be processed as standard.

Waste

This should be treated as clinical waste.

Linen

Treat as infected.

Transfers to other wards and departments
There are no restrictions on ward transfers if for clinical reasons.

Visits to other departments, such as radiology, should be kept to a minimum. Where visits are necessary the receiving department must be told in advance and the following principles applied:

- Transporting staff, for example porters, should wear disposable gloves and aprons only when they are in contact with the patient; these should be discarded immediately contact has ceased.
- Transporting staff do not need to wear masks.
- Hand hygiene by hand washing or alcohol gel is necessary after patient and equipment contact.
- Trolleys or wheelchairs used for patient transfers should be decontaminated before use on another patient.
- Patients should not wait in holding areas with other patients, wherever possible, but should be brought to the department immediately before and returned to their isolation room immediately after treatments or investigations.

Visitors
There is no restriction on visitors. Protective clothing (gloves and aprons) need only be worn when carrying out bodily care activities. All visitors should be instructed on the precautions required, including hand hygiene on leaving the room.

Close relatives and household contacts may be given antibiotic prophylaxis; this is sometimes dispensed from ward stock.

Deceased patients
Last offices should be performed as standard practice. A body bag should be used and the mortuary advised in advance.

MULTI-RESISTANT GRAM NEGATIVE BACTERIA (ESBLS)
Extended-spectrum β-lactamases are a group of enzymes that make some Gram negative bacteria (e.g. enterobacters, *Klebsiella* spp., *Escherichia coli*) resistant to a number of antibiotic groups,

including penicillins and cephalosporins. They are generally found in the gastro-intestinal tract and cause any infection commonly associated with Gram negative bacteria, including urine infections and wound infections. Risk factors for colonisation and infection include:

- Prolonged hospital stay
- Prolonged stay in an intensive care unit
- Presence of an invasive device
- Repeated courses of antibiotics

Outbreaks of infection have been reported in the community as well as in hospital settings (Pelly *et al.*, 2006), with practice during clinical procedures and contaminated equipment implicated in outbreaks (Rogues *et al.*, 2000). Spread of contamination by healthcare workers' hands is considered to be one of the key routes of transmission (International Infection Control Council, 2005).

Limiting the use of antibiotics is important in prevention of infection. In addition to standard precautions, the following additional precautions are often applied (International Infection Control Council, 2005; Department of Health, Social Services and Public Safety, 2006).

Patient placement
Single room isolation is preferable, particularly in critical care areas. If patients with ESBLs are to remain on general wards then care should be taken that they are not placed in proximity to patients with risk factors for ESBL carriage, for example patients with an indwelling urethral catheter.

Discontinuation of isolation
Testing for clearance of ESBL may be helpful in determining when isolation can be discontinued. Three consecutive negative specimens, taken a week apart, from known colonised and infected sites have been suggested as the criteria for discontinuation of isolation. As discontinuation of isolation can depend on a variety of factors, advice should be sought from the infection control team.

Staff

There is no restriction on staff.

Visiting staff, for example physiotherapists, should be given instructions on precautions that are required before they enter the room.

Treatment

Patients with infections will be treated systemically with appropriate antibiotics. Treatment of colonisation is not generally indicated as this may encourage further antibiotic resistance to develop.

Protective clothing

- Gloves should be worn for all contact with the patient and their immediate environment.
- Aprons should be worn by all staff who will be handling the patient or who will have contact with their immediate environment, for example cleaning staff.
- Masks are generally not required but should be worn when a risk assessment under standard precautions dictates.

Hand hygiene

Hands should be decontaminated by either hand washing or the use of an alcohol gel before and after contact with the patient or their immediate environment.

Cleaning procedures

General cleaning

A good standard of general cleaning on a daily basis is required. Detergent and water is sufficient; however, a disinfectant, for example hypochlorite, may be used.

Discharge cleaning

The room should undergo a thorough and enhanced clean to include areas where dust may collect, including radiators and ventilator ducts. A disinfectant, for example hypochlorite, should be used. Curtains should be removed and laundered.

Equipment
Where possible, equipment should be single use or dedicated for the individual patient's use. Reusable equipment must be adequately decontaminated before using on another patient (refer to Chapter 16).

Crockery and cutlery may be washed in the dishwasher in the usual manner.

Waste
All waste should be discarded as clinical waste.

Linen
All linen should be treated as infected.

Transfers to other wards and departments
Patients should not be transferred to other wards until it is clinically necessary.

Visits to other departments, such as radiology, should be kept to a minimum. Where visits are necessary the receiving department must be told in advance and the following principles applied:

- Transporting staff, for example porters, should wear disposable gloves and aprons only when they are in contact with the patient; these should be discarded immediately contact has ceased.
- Hand hygiene by hand washing or alcohol gel is necessary after patient and equipment contact.
- Trolleys or wheelchairs used for patient transfers should be decontaminated before use on another patient.
- Patients should not wait in holding areas with other patients, wherever possible, but should be brought to the department immediately before and returned to their isolation room immediately after treatments or investigations.

Visitors

There is no restriction on visitors. Protective clothing (gloves and aprons) need only be worn when carrying out bodily care activities. All visitors should be instructed on the precautions required, including hand hygiene on leaving the room.

Discharge

ESBL carriage should not delay a patient's discharge if they are medically fit. The GP and/or district nurse should be informed of the patient's ESBL status. The following information will be required:

- Date and site of initial ESBL positive specimen (if during this admission)
- Details of any actual infection
- Date and results of most recent ESBL screen if applicable

Patients and carers should be advised that there are no specific restrictions or precautions needed for patients being discharged to their own home. Patients should be advised that if they require further hospitalisation or healthcare treatments then they should inform staff prior to treatment, wherever possible, that they have been ESBL positive.

Ambulance staff should be informed in advance. There is generally no restriction on ambulance transport; however, ESBL positive patients should not be transported with other patients who may be more susceptible, such as those with indwelling urinary catheters.

Deceased patients

No specific precautions are required.

NOROVIRUS

Norovirus is a common cause of outbreaks of gastroenteritis in hospitals. It is also commonly referred to as norwalk virus, winter vomiting disease, or small, round, structured virus. It causes acute gastroenteritis that lasts 12–60 hours, affecting all ages. Diarrhoea and/or vomiting can occur, but instances of vomiting are generally greater with norovirus than with other viral causes of gastroenteritis. Outbreaks of infection also occur outside hospitals, often in schools, nurseries, hotels and on cruise ships. Transmission is by the faecal-oral route, aerosols of vomit, food, or water borne. Only a small number of virus particles are needed to cause infection, making it highly transmissible in wards. Signs and symptoms include diarrhoea, vomiting, nausea, general malaise, stomach cramps, pyrexia and headaches. The incubation period can be as short as 12 hours but up to 48 hours. The virus is excreted in stools for several days after cessation of symptoms. There is a short-lived immunity after infection but as there can be different strains of the virus in circulation at any one time, immunity is not assured. Specimens of vomit or faeces are examined microscopically as well as undergoing molecular testing. Norovirus infection does not generally require hospitalisation and it is rarely fatal; however, the dehydration associated with diarrhoea and vomiting can lead to an exacerbation of underlying medical conditions, making hospitalisation necessary.

Management of individual cases

Patient placement

- Patients admitted with suspected norovirus or other viral gastroenteritis should be admitted to a single room.
- En suite facilities should be available wherever possible.
- The door should be kept closed at all times.

Staff

- A limited number of staff should care for the patient.
- Visiting staff, for example physiotherapists, should not see symptomatic patients unless clinically necessary.
- Visiting staff should see patients with suspected or confirmed infection at the end of their schedule.

Treatment

- There is no active treatment; supportive therapy, for example fluid replacement, is recommended in line with the patient's clinical condition.

- The administration of anti-emetics may be beneficial in preventing airborne spread in vomiting patients.

Protective clothing

Staff entering the single room should wear gloves and aprons for direct patient contact and for contact with the patient's immediate environment, for example cleaning.

Hand hygiene

- All staff and visitors entering the room should wash their hands with soap and water before entering and on leaving the room.
- Alcohol hand gels can have limited efficiency with some gastro-intestinal viruses.

Cleaning procedures

- The patient's room should be cleaned daily, paying particular attention to sanitary equipment, for example toilets.
- A disinfectant, for example hypochlorite, should be used for all cleaning.

Discharge cleaning

The room should undergo a thorough and enhanced clean, particularly for sanitary equipment. A disinfectant, for example hypochlorite, should be used. Curtains should be removed and laundered.

Equipment

Where possible, equipment should be single use or dedicated for the individual patient's use. Reusable equipment must be adequately decontaminated before using on another patient (refer to Chapter 16).

Crockery and cutlery may be washed in the dishwasher in the usual manner.

Waste

All waste should be discarded as clinical waste.

Linen
All linen should be treated as infected.

Transfers to other wards and departments
Patients with confirmed or suspected norovirus who are symptomatic should not be transferred to other wards until it is clinically necessary. The receiving ward should be informed in advance and should be advised that single room isolation is necessary.

Visits to other departments, such as radiology, should be kept to a minimum and avoided if patients are symptomatic with diarrhoea and/or vomiting, unless clinically essential. Where visits are necessary the receiving department must be told in advance and the following principles applied:

- Transporting staff, for example porters, should wear disposable gloves and aprons only when they are in contact with the patient; these should be discarded immediately contact has ceased.
- Hand hygiene by hand washing is necessary after patient and equipment contact.
- Trolleys or wheelchairs used for patient transfers should be decontaminated before use on another patient.
- Patients must not wait in holding areas with other patients; they should be brought to the department immediately before and returned to their isolation room immediately after treatments or investigations.

Visitors
Visiting should be discouraged if patients are symptomatic. Visitors who themselves are symptomatic with diarrhoea and/or vomiting should not visit.

Protective clothing (gloves and aprons) need only be worn when carrying out bodily care activities. All visitors should be instructed on the precautions required, including hand washing on leaving the room.

Discharge
If patients are being discharged to nursing or residential care then the home should be contacted in advance. It may be necessary to

delay discharge until the patient is asymptomatic to reduce the risk of infection spreading in that care setting.

Deceased patients
No specific precautions are required.

Additional actions in event of a ward outbreak

- The ward should be closed to all new admissions.
- Only essential staff should enter the ward area.
- Agency and bank staff should not be used.
- Symptomatic staff should go off duty immediately.
- Food and drink should not be consumed in patient areas.
- Exposed food, such as patient's fruit, should be discarded.
- The frequency of cleaning should be increased, with sanitary equipment cleaned twice daily as a minimum.
- Air currents should be kept to a minimum to reduce airborne spread. Windows should be kept closed and fans should not be used.
- The ward should not be re-opened until 72 hours have elapsed from the last new case amongst staff or patients.

SCENARIO

Mr Phillips is a 72-year-old gentleman who has been admitted to hospital with an exacerbation of chronic obstructive airways disease. A sputum specimen sent to the laboratory has shown the presence of MRSA, and screening swabs show that it is also in his nose. What are the infection control precautions that should now be taken?

Mr Phillips should be moved to a single room. Both he and his family should be advised of the presence of MRSA and the precautions that will now be taken. Staff should wear gloves and aprons for all patient contact and when handling potentially contaminated equipment in the room. The room should be cleaned at least daily, taking care not to create dust. Mr Phillips should be given a course of topical decolonisation therapy. Clinical equipment, for example commode and blood pressure monitors, should be dedicated to use in his room alone and should be adequately decontaminated before use on any other patient. Waste should be discarded as clinical waste and linen handled as infected, in line with local policy.

- The ward should be thoroughly cleaned with a disinfectant, for example hypochlorite, and all curtains changed before re-opening. (Chadwick *et al.*, 2000)

SUMMARY
In addition to standard infection control principles, additional precautions may be needed for patients with specific infections in hospitals. The additional precautions for MRSA, *Clostridium difficile*, GRE, norovirus, multi-resistant Gram negative bacteria, Creutzfeldt-Jakob disease, meningococcal meningitis and tuberculosis have been outlined. Application of these additional precautions is essential to prevent the spread of important pathogens in hospital settings.

REFERENCES
Advisory Committee on Dangerous Pathogens and the Spongiform Encephalopathy Advisory Committee (2003) *Transmissible Spongiform Encephalopathy Agents: Safe Working and the Prevention of Infection.* Available at: http://www.advisorybodies.doh.gov.uk/acdp/tseguidance/Index.htm (accessed on 25 November 2006).

Ayliffe, G.A.J., Buckles, A., Casewell, M.W *et al.* (1998) Revised guidelines for the control of meticillin resistant *Staphylococcus aureus* infection in hospitals. *Journal of Hospital Infection*, **39** (4), 253–290.

Barnett, J., Thomlinson, D., Perry, C., Marshall, R. and MacGowan, A.P. (1999) An audit of the use of manual handling equipment and their microbiological flora – implications for infection control. *Journal of Hospital Infection*, **43** (4), 309–313.

Bolyard, E.A., Tablan, O.C., Williams, W.W., Pearson, M.L., Shapiro, C.N., Deitchman, S.D., and the Hospital Infection Control Practices Advisory Committee (1998) Guideline for infection control in healthcare personnel. *American Journal of Infection Control*, **26**, 289–354.

Bradley, C. and Fraise, A.P. (1996) Heat and chemical resistance of enterococci. *Journal of Hospital Infection*, **34** (3), 191–196.

British Thoracic Society (2000) Control and prevention of tuberculosis in the United Kingdom: code of practice 2000. Joint Tuberculosis Committee of the British Thoracic Society. *Thorax*, **55** (11), 887–901.

Centers for Disease Control and Prevention (1995) Recommendations for preventing the spread of vancomycin resistance: recommendations of the Hospital Infection Control Practices Advisory Committee (HICPAC). *Mortality and Morbidity Weekly Report*, **44**, 1–13.

Chadwick, P.R., Beards, G., Brown, E. *et al.* (2000) Management of hospital outbreaks of gastroenteritis due to small, round structured viruses: report of the public health laboratory service viral gastro-enteritis working group. *Journal of Hospital Infection*, **45** (1), 1–10.

Coia, J.E., Duckworth, G.K., Edwards, D.I., *et al.* (2006) Guidelines for the control and prevention of meticillin resistant *Staphylococcus aureus* (MRSA) in healthcare facilities. *Journal of Hospital Infection*, **63** (suppl.), s1–44.

Cookson, B.D., Macrea, M.B., Barrett, S.P. *et al.* (2006) Guidelines for the control of glycopeptide resistant enterococci in hospitals. *Journal of Hospital Infection*, **62** (1), 6–21.

Das, I. and Jumaa, P. (2006) Has the severity of *Clostridium difficile* infections increased? *Journal of Hospital Infection*, **65** (1), 85–86.

Department of Health (2004) *Stopping Tuberculosis in England: an Action Plan from the Chief Medical Officer*. Department of Health, London.

Department of Health (2006) Screening for meticillin resistant *Staphylococcus aureus* (MRSA) colonisation: a strategy for NHS trusts – a summary of best practice. Available at: http://www.dh.gov.uk/en/Publicationsandstatistics/Publications/PublicationsPolicyAndGuidance/DH_063188 (accessed 10 April 2007).

Department of Health (undated) *Creutzfeldt-Jakob Disease: Guidance for Healthcare Workers*. Available at: http://www.dh.gov.uk/assetRoot/04/08/23/70/04082370.pdf (accessed 25 November 2006).

Department of Health and Public Health Laboratory Service (1994) *Clostridium difficile Infection: Prevention and Management*. Department of Health, London.

Department of Health, Social Services and Public Safety (2006) *Guidance on Patients with Extended-spectrum β-lactamase (ESBL) Producing Gram-Negative Bacteria*. Available at: http://www.dhsspsni.gov.uk/ph_esbl.pdf (accessed 25 November 2006).

Fekety, R., Kim, K.H., Brown, D., Batts, D.H., Cudmore, M. and Silva, J. (1981) Epidemiology of antibiotic associated colitis: isolation of *Clostridium difficile* from the hospital environment. *American Medical Journal*, **70**, 906–908.

Health Protection Agency (2006a) *Surveillance of Surgical Site Infection in England: October 1997–September 2005*. Health Protection Agency, London.

Health Protection Agency (2006b) *Voluntary Surveillance of Clostridium difficile Associated Disease in England, Wales and Northern Ireland, 2005*. Available at: http://www.hpa.org.uk/infections/topics_az/clostridium_difficile/C_difficile_Voluntary_Report_2006.pdf (accessed 25 November 2006).

International Infection Control Council (2005) *Best Infection Control Practices for Patients with Extended Spectrum Beta-lactamase Enterobacteriacae*. Available at: www.icna.co.uk. (accessed 20 November 2006).

Joint Tuberculosis Committee of the British Thoracic Society (2000) Control and prevention of tuberculosis in the United Kingdom: Code of Practice. *Thorax*, **55** (11), 887–901.

Kent, R.J., Uttley, A.H.C., Stoker, N.G., Miller, R. and Pozniak, A.L. (1994) Transmission of tuberculosis in a British care centre for patients infected with HIV. *British Medical Journal*, **309**, 639–640.

Manian, F.A., Meyer, L. and Jenne, J. (1996) *Clostridium difficile* contamination of blood pressure cuffs: a call for a closer look at gloving practices in the era of universal precautions. *Infection Control and Hospital Epidemiology*, **17** (3), 180–182.

Murray, B.E. (1990) The life and times of the enterococcus. *Clinical Microbiology Reviews*, **3**, 46–65.

Pelly, H., Morris, D., O'Connell, E. *et al.* (2006) Outbreak of an extended spectrum beta-lactamase producing *E. coli* in a nursing home in Ireland, May 2006. *Eurosurveillance Weekly*, **11** (8).

Public Health Laboratory Service (2002) Guidelines for public health management of meningococcal disease in the UK. *Communicable Disease and Public Health*, **5** (3), 187–204.

Rogues, A.M., Boulard, G., Allery, A. *et al.* (2000) Thermometers as a vehicle for transmission of extended-spectrum-β-lactamase producing *Klebsiella pneumoniae*. *Journal of Hospital Infection*, **45** (1), 77–78.

Royal College of Physicians (2006) *Tuberculosis: Clinical Diagnosis and Management of Tuberculosis and Measures for its Prevention and Control*. Royal College of Physicians, London.

The Interdepartmental Working Group on Tuberculosis (1996) *The Prevention and Control of Tuberculosis in the United Kingdom: Recommendations for the Prevention and Control of Tuberculosis at Local Level*. Department of Health, London.

The Interdepartmental Working Group on Tuberculosis (1998) *The Prevention and Control of Tuberculosis in the United Kingdom: UK Guidance on the Prevention and Control of (1) HIV-related Tuberculosis and (2) Drug-resistant including Multiple Drug-resistant Tuberculosis*. Department of Health, London.

Wilcox, M. (2003) *Antibiotics and Clostridium difficile Infection* (third edition) Eurocommunica Limited, Barnham.

7 | Infection Prevention in Urinary Catheter Care

Lauren Tew

INTRODUCTION

Healthcare is now providing more advanced therapies for more acutely ill and older people than ever before. This patient population will increasingly need the therapeutic facilities associated with urinary catheterisation. Urinary catheters drain urine from the bladder for a wide range of purposes, from acute accurate measurement of urine volumes to chronic management of intractable urinary incontinence. All invasive medical procedures are associated with infection risks (see also Chapter 8, Infection Prevention in Intravascular Therapy) and contemporary healthcare professionals need to be competent and confident in this aspect of care in order to reduce these risks.

LEARNING OBJECTIVES

By the end of this chapter you will be able to:

❏ Identify infection prevention principles relating to urinary catheters
❏ Discuss the role of biofilms in the process of catheter associated urinary tract infection (CAUTI)
❏ Describe the routes by which micro-organisms causing CAUTI gain access
❏ List factors increasing patients' risk of CAUTI
❏ Summarise contemporary evidence based guidelines to reduce infection risks

It has been estimated that 25% of patients admitted to hospital will be catheterised (Bandolier, 1998), but this does not mean that the procedure is without risk (Tew *et al.*, 2005). Catheter associated urinary tract infection (CAUTI) is the most frequent and probably most easily preventable healthcare associated infection worldwide (Salgado *et al.*, 2003; Tambyah, 2004). Definitions of CAUTI can vary. Some studies use a definition based on microbiological evidence only, whilst others insist on evidence of clinical symptoms also. The recent UK prevalence survey of healthcare associated infections used definitions that demand both microbiological and symptomatic evidence of infection. Symptoms of CAUTI will include, for example, fever, dysuria and suprapubic tenderness (Horan and Gaynes, 2004). Bacteria will be found in urine in the majority of cases within a few days of catheterisation. This is known as asymptomatic bacteriuria and, of itself, does not indicate infection and will often resolve quickly once the catheter is removed. Once symptoms appear, that is symptomatic bacteriuria, these indicate that an infection has developed.

Urinary catheters can be of the self-retaining type (Foley) draining urine continually, or can be used to drain the bladder intermittently; they can be for short or long-term use and can be manufactured from a variety of materials. Foley/indwelling catheters are held in place in the bladder with a small balloon inflated with sterile water. Urethral or suprapubic routes into the bladder may be chosen. Other characteristics include their diameter, their length and the volume of the retaining balloon. A full description of the assessment process to determine which type of urinary catheter will best suit the individual patient is beyond the remit of this chapter. Healthcare providers should have local policies available to guide practitioners' choice, compiled by collaboration between relevant experts, such as infection prevention and control practitioners, continence advisors and urology nurse specialists (Pomfret *et al.*, 2006).

INFECTION PREVENTION PRINCIPLES
There are two fundamental principles underpinning all other infection prevention activity with regard to urinary catheterisation:

(1) Only catheterise when absolutely essential.
(2) Remove urinary catheters as soon as possible.

Only catheterise when absolutely essential

There are occasions when patients are catheterised without due justification and consideration of the risks involved (Saint *et al.*, 2002). Death from bacteraemia can ensue as a direct result of urinary catheterisation. This is relatively rare, but urinary catheterisation does place the patient at *significant danger* (Pratt *et al.*, 2007) of urinary tract infection and this risk must be borne in mind when this invasive procedure is considered.

Always consider other alternatives, such as external devices, before placing an indwelling urinary catheter. Thoroughly document the rationale behind the decision to catheterise in the patient's health records.

Indications for catheterisation (based on Pomfret, 1999) are:

- Relief of urinary tract obstruction and retention of urine
- Enlarged prostate gland
- Drainage of the bladder when its muscles or nerves are not working properly
- Before and after pelvic surgery
- To accurately measure urinary output, for example in intensive care units
- To obtain an uncontaminated specimen of urine
- To empty the bladder during labour
- To irrigate the bladder
- Administration of therapies and treatments
- Investigation of urinary tract function
- Management of urinary incontinence when all other methods are not applicable

Remove urinary catheters as soon as possible

If urinary catheterisation is deemed to be essential, an effective way to reduce infection risks is to remove the catheter at the earliest opportunity. Prolonged catheterisation has been identified as the greatest risk factor for CAUTI (Maki and Tambyah, 2001). When completing documentation regarding the catheterisation process, always ensure that review of the necessity for the catheter is planned; early removal is likely to reduce CAUTI rates (Saint *et al.*, 2005)

ROLE OF BIOFILMS

An understanding of the role of biofilms in the development of CAUTI is essential as they influence every aspect of CAUTI, from its cause, diagnosis and treatment (Trauntner and Darouiche, 2004). Biofilms, which are communities of micro-organisms and their extracellular products (Tenke *et al.*, 2004) and can be found on the catheter, the drainage system and the uroepithelium lining the urinary tract, are a basic survival strategy for micro-organisms and can be described as the 'high rise, des res, gated communities' of the microbial world:

- **High rise**

  — An initial 'ground floor' of conditioning film settles on the surface of the urinary catheter. This will comprise urinary proteins and micro-organisms. No surface has yet been designed that will resist biofilm development entirely, although much research is in progress. Some surfaces, for example silver alloy coating, have been shown to reduce biofilm adherence.

  — Once a conditioning layer is in place, a biofilm matrix forms, onto which bacteria will settle.

  — Whilst some biofilm colonies are single layer and patchy, others develop into several layers deep and cover the catheter surface completely (Ganderton *et al.*, 1992)

- **Des res**

  — Some bacteria will remain in the free-floating (planktonic) state, but others will settle within the biofilm matrix.

  — Some biofilms are made up of a single species of bacteria, but most attract up to four.

- **Gated communities**

  — Bacteria in biofilm communities show exclusive characteristics that differ from their planktonic form.

  — For example, biofilm bacteria are up to 1000 times more resistant to antibiotics than their free-floating types (Tenke *et al.*, 2004).

— The close relationship between bacterial families in biofilms promotes the exchange of resistance to antimicrobial agents.

ROUTES OF INFECTION

The two main routes by which micro-organisms gain access to the catheterised urinary tract are described below:

• **Extra-luminal**

This route is via the exterior surface of the urinary catheter, from its contact with the organisms on the skin around the entrance of the catheter into the body, the urethral meatus. This route predominates in females. The proximity of the urethral meatus to the perineum and anus facilitates contamination from skin organisms, such as *Staphylococcus aureus*. Careful insertion to avoid inoculation of micro-organisms into the bladder, aseptic technique and maintenance of the patient's personal hygiene will all contribute to reducing this risk.

• **Intra-luminal**

The internal surface of the urinary catheter provides the intra-luminal route. This route affects male patients particularly. It is caused by unhygienic management and handling of the urinary catheter and its drainage system. For example, the outlet port of the collection bag may be contaminated when emptying it into a vessel that has not been adequately decontaminated. Infections transmitted by this route are caused by such organisms as *Escherichia coli* and *Pseudomonas aeruginosa* (Donlan, 2001).

RISK FACTORS

There are certain factors that increase the risk of a patient developing a urinary tract infection associated with their catheter. These include:

• Prolonged catheterisation, more than six days
• Female gender
• Other infections
• Diabetes
• Malnutrition

- Renal failure
- Drainage tube above level of bladder
- Microbial virulence factors
- Older age (from Salgado *et al.*, 2003; Tambyah, 2004)

By reviewing these it is clear that many patients receiving healthcare will have some, if not many, risk factors. Such awareness is the first step in the prevention of CAUTI. The next step is to implement evidence based guidelines to reduce these risks.

EVIDENCE BASED GUIDELINES
The Department of Health has commissioned the writing and review of evidence based guidelines for the prevention of infection in both hospital and community settings (Pratt *et al.*, 2007). Those referring to the care of patients with urinary catheters are given in Table 7.1, below.

CATHETERISATION PROCEDURE
As already mentioned, urinary catheterisation is a skilled procedure. Healthcare practitioners must be trained in the technique and competent in its performance. Mangnall and Watterson (2006) describe aseptic techniques as those practices that reduce the risk of the patient developing an infection after the procedure by decreasing the possibility of micro-organisms entering the body during the procedure. Table 7.2 identifies some useful tips when performing urethral catheterisation.

Suprapubic catheterisation
Suprapubic catheterisation involves inserting the catheter into the bladder through the abdominal wall and is usually reserved for those patients needing catheterisation in the long term. The initial insertion is usually undertaken by medical staff, but competent nursing staff may undertake subsequent replacements. It is associated with less risk of infection than indwelling urethral catheterisation. Once healed, the small abdominal opening may need only routine hygiene to be kept clean. Sometimes infection with micro-organisms living on the skin (such as *S. aureus*) can need treatment and dressing (see Chapter 10). Urinary stones can occasionally complicate the health of patients with suprapubic catheters and may be found when CAUTIs recur.

Table 7.1 Evidence based guidelines for the prevention of catheter-associated urinary tract infections.

Guidelines	Rationale
• Catheterise only if absolutely necessary. • Review need for catheterisation regularly. • Remove catheter as soon as possible.	These first, fundamental principles have been discussed above and form the basis for sound infection prevention practice for catheterised patients. The following guidelines must also be applied for safe management of the catheterised patient.
• Trained, competent staff to insert, change and maintain catheters aseptically.	Catheterisation and the management of indwelling catheters are skilled procedures that require appropriate training.
• Select smallest gauge to allow free flow of urine.	The urethra is normally closed except when urine is voided. A catheter holds it artificially open and, if too large in diameter, can cause damage to the delicate tissues lining the urethra and blocking para-urethral glands, predisposing these tissues to infection. A size 12 Fg is suitable for both men and women draining clear urine. Large sizes may be needed for urine containing debris. Patients who have undergone urological surgery may need larger catheters to allow for the drainage of blood clots.
• Assessment will consider clinical need, anticipated duration, patient preference, and infection risk.	There is no 'one size fits all' when it comes to urinary catheters.
• Use silver alloy hydrogel coated catheters appropriately.	There is evidence that silver alloy coated catheters are effective in reducing CAUTI in the patient groups that have been studied (Brosnahan et al., 2004). The Department of Health's Rapid Review Panel (2004) has recommended that these be available for use within the NHS. Some trusts have converted to these as their catheter of choice in order to reduce CAUTI.
• Use lubricant from single-use container.	Lubricant should be used for both male and female catheterisation in order to reduce urethral trauma on insertion of the catheter, thus reducing infection risk. A single use container removes the risk of transmission of microbial contamination between patients.

Table 7.1 *Continued*

Guidelines	Rationale
• Use 10 ml balloon for adults, 3–5 ml for children (unless necessary for urological purposes).	The Foley indwelling catheter is held in place by inflating a small balloon that prevents the catheter from sliding back down the urethra after insertion into the bladder. The eyes of the catheter are above the balloon, causing a residual amount of urine to remain within the bladder. Using a 10 ml balloon reduces this ideal environment for microbial multiplication to a minimum.
• Document insertion, changes and care in individual catheter care regimen.	Accurate documentation will facilitate appropriate care, for example by ensuring catheter changes are undertaken appropriately.
• Decontaminate hands and wear gloves for any manipulation of the system.	This will ensure that the risk of transmission of micro-organisms between patients or from the health care practitioner to the patient is minimised.
• Decontaminate hands after removing gloves.	Gloves are no substitute for hand hygiene and can have micro-perforations through which contamination may occur.
• Ensure gravity drainage, positioning drainage bags below the bladder and off the floor.	Urine cannot flow up hill, but will stagnate in the bladder if gravity drainage is not allowed. Back flow into the bladder by lifting the bag above the bladder must be avoided – non-return valves are no barrier to micro-organisms.
• Daily meatal hygiene with soap and water and prior to catheter insertion.	There is no evidence that daily cleansing with antiseptics reduces CAUTI rates. It may encourage antimicrobial resistance.
• The catheter and drainage system should not be disconnected except for good clinical reasons; use a link system overnight.	Every time a urinary catheter is detached from its drainage system this provides an opportunity for microbial contamination. Attach a link system to the drainage system, without disconnecting the urinary catheter, to increase the urine reservoir volume overnight.
• Don't change catheters or empty drainage bags routinely but when clinically indicated. Follow manufacturer's instructions.	In the UK and Europe most catheters are licensed either for 28 days or 12 weeks use and must be changed at that time, if not before. If a healthcare practitioner decides to leave a urinary catheter in place for longer than its licence permits, the liability for the functioning of that catheter moves to that practitioner and away from the manufacturer.

Table 7.1 *Continued*

Guidelines	Rationale
• Sample aseptically.	This will avoid contamination of the system.
• Monitor tendency to blockage.	Some people who are catheterised for the long term have a tendency to form encrustations that block the catheter completely. By monitoring and documenting this a pattern may become clear and steps can be taken to avoid the distress and danger to the patient of a complete blockage of their catheter.
• Irrigations, instillations and washouts do not prevent infection.	Such procedures should not be undertaken routinely but only as a planned regime of care for an individual patient for whom their use is beneficial.
• Training and support should be available for patients with long-term catheters and their carers.	Patients and carers who use urinary catheters in the long term need to understand the function of the catheter. They also need to know basic hygiene and trouble-shooting strategies, and who to contact when problems arise.
• Consider intermittent catheterization.	The passage of a catheter at regular intervals to empty the bladder, and then its removal, is associated with less risk of infection than either suprapubic (through the abdominal wall) or urethral routes, but is dependent on the patient's mental and manual dexterity. Sometimes a carer will undertake this function.
• Consider the use of a catheter valve.	A catheter valve can be used to empty the bladder periodically, so maintaining the tone of the bladder muscles. This can be a useful option for those patients who have the necessary mental and manual dexterity and reduces the risk of transmission of micro-organisms from carer's hands.
• Avoid antibiotic prophylaxis unless clinically indicated.	Patients with long-term catheters are more likely to be colonised with antimicrobial resistant micro-organisms as a result of repeated prescriptions for antibiotics. This, together with the proximity of resistant organisms living in the biofilms on urinary drainage systems, facilitates the spread of resistance between species. Prophylaxis should only be given in specific circumstances as described in the National Institute for Audit and Clinical Excellence Guidelines (see NICE, 2003) and in consultation with the local consultant medical microbiologist.

Table 7.1 *Continued*

Guidelines	Rationale
• Reusable intermittent catheters should be cleaned with water and stored dry in accordance with manufacturers' instructions.	Some people using catheters intermittently prefer the reusable to the disposable, single use type.

(Above guidelines based on Pratt *et al.*, 2007; NICE, 2003; Pellowe *et al.*, 2004).

Table 7.2 Top tips for catheterisation procedure.

Do	Don't
☑ Have a colleague at hand to assist you whenever you can	☒ Forget to explain to the patient what's going to happen to a very private part of their anatomy
☑ Follow local policy comprehensively	☒ Omit to document all details of the procedure, including the fact that the patient has agreed to it
☑ Ensure a good light source, especially when catheterising a female	☒ Allow the drainage tap to drag on the floor
☑ Perform aseptic technique scrupulously	☒ Let loops of drainage tubing hang down below the drainage bag
☑ When catheterising a female, leave a misplaced catheter (i.e. in the vagina) until you have placed a catheter in the urethra, to ensure the same mistake doesn't happen again	☒ Reuse a misplaced contaminated catheter – always use a sterile one
☑ Attach the drainage system before inserting the catheter	☒ Use any other solution to inflate the balloon than sterile water
☑ Use lubrication for both men and women	

Long-term catheterisation

Prevention of CAUTI in some patients who need to live with their catheter in place in the long term can be difficult to achieve. Bacteria will colonise the long-term catheterised urinary tract (bacteriuria) and inflammation will be indicated by pus cells in the urine (pyuria). Both bacteriuria and pyuria can be found at surprisingly high levels in those with long-term catheters, and are not diagnostic of infection (Nicolle, 2001). This group of patients may well be elderly, and conventional definitions of CAUTI, which are appropriate for those catheterised for the short term, may be difficult to apply. Pyrexia may not occur, but a change in mental faculties, such as confusion, may be indicative of illness. Strict adherence to the principles of infection prevention must still be applied to this group of patients.

Encrustation and blockage of the urinary catheter is a problem for about half of chronically catheterised patients. A complex cascade of biochemical events, beginning with colonisation with urease producing micro-organisms such as *Proteus mirabilis,* can end with crystals precipitating out of the patient's urine and, together with the biofilm matrix, blocking the drainage of urine entirely (Morris and Stickler, 1998; Mathur *et al.*, 2006). Compliance

---

SCENARIO

An elderly lady with renal failure, Mrs Underhill, has arrived on your ward from the admissions unit with a Foley catheter in place. What information will you seek immediately to inform your care for her?

All of the following need to be considered in order to reduce Mrs Underhill's risk of CAUTI:

- What is Mrs Underhill's condition now, and is she comfortable?
- Why was Mrs Underhill catheterised?
- Is Mrs Underhill's urine draining freely into a drainage bag that is below her bladder and off the floor?
- Are all the details of the procedure, the catheter and the drainage system documented?
- When will the need for the catheter be reviewed?
- What does Mrs Underhill understand about her catheter and hygiene needs?

---

with infection prevention precautions must be complete when interventions such as changing the catheter are undertaken. Every breakage of the closed system, by disconnecting the catheter from its drainage tube, is an opportunity for contamination with and transmission of micro-organisms. Efforts to pre-empt future blockage will include accurate documentation of, for example, a catheter diary which may indicate a trend to block after a certain time.

SUMMARY

The presence of an indwelling urinary catheter places patients at significant risk of infection. Bacteria can be found in the urine of catheterised patients within a few days of catheterisation. Urinary tract infection can lead to more serious infection, including bacteraemia. Avoiding insertion and removing urinary catheters are important infection prevention strategies. Aseptic technique for insertion and management of urinary catheters is one of the most important aspects of catheter care.

REFERENCES

Association for Continence Advice (2007) *Notes on Good Practice*. Updated 2007 (online). Association for Continence Advice. Available at: http://www.notesongoodpractice.co.uk/ (accessed 12 January 2007).

Bandolier, (1998) Urinary catheters. Dec., 58–3. Available at: http://www.jr2.ox.ac.uk/bandolier/band58/b58-3.html (accessed 12 January 2007).

BARD (2003) *Indwelling Catheters: Integrated Care Pathway Package*. Harvard Health, Surrey, UK.

Brosnahan, J., Jull, A. and Tracy, C. (2004) Types of urethral catheters for management of short-term voiding problems in hospitalised adults (Cochrane Review) In: *The Cochrane Library*, **1**. John Wiley & Sons Ltd, Chichester.

Department of Health (2004) *Rapid Review Panel Report*. Available at: http://www.hpa.org.uk/infections/topics_az/rapid_review/pdf/bardex2.pdf (accessed 12 January 2007).

Donlan, R. (2001) Biofilms and device associated infections. *Emerging Infectious Diseases*, **7** (2). Available at: http://www.cdc.gov/ncidod/eid/vol7no2/donlan.htm (accessed 12 January 2007).

Ganderton, L., Chawla, J., Winters, C., Wimpenny, J. and Stickler, D. (1992) Scanning electron microscopy of bacterial biofilms on indwelling bladder catheters *European Journal of Clinical Microbiology and Infectious Diseases*, September, 789–796.

Horan, T.C. and Gaynes, R.P. (2004) Surveillance of nosocomial infections. In: *Hospital Epidemiology and Infection Control* (ed. C.G. Mayhall), (third edition). Lippincott Williams & Wilkins, Philadelphia.

Maki, D. and Tambyah, P. (2001) Engineering out the risk of infection with urinary catheters. *Emerging Infectious Diseases*, **7** (2), 1–6.

Mangnall, J. and Watterson, L. (2006) Principles of aseptic technique in urinary catheterisation. *Nursing Standard*, **21** (8), 49–56.

Mathur, S., Suller, M.T.E., Stickler, D. and Feneley, R. (2006) Prospective study of individuals with long-term urinary catheters colonised with proteus species. *BJU International*, **97**, 121–128.

Morris, N.S. and Stickler, D.J. (1998) Encrustation of indwelling urethral catheters by *Proteus mirabilis* biofilms growing in human urine. *Journal of Hospital Infection*, **39**, 227–234.

National Institute for Clinical Excellence (2003) *Full Guideline: Prevention of Healthcare Associated Infection in Primary and Community Care, Section 3 – Urinary Catheterisation.* Available at: http://www.nice.org.uk/guidance/CG2 (accessed 12 January 2007).

Nicolle, L. (2001) Urinary tract infections in long-term care facilities. *Infection Control and Hospital Epidemiology*, **22** (3), 167–175.

Pellowe, C.M., Pratt, R.J., Loveday, H.P., Harper, P., Robinson, N. and Jones, S.R.L.J. (2004) The *epic* project. Updating the evidence base for national evidence based guidelines for preventing healthcare associated infections in NHS hospitals in England: a report with recommendations. *British Journal of Infection Control*, **5** (6), 10–16.

Pomfret, I. (1999) Catheter care. *Primary Health Care*, **9** (5), 29–36.

Pomfret, I., Holden, C., King, D. *et al.* (2006) Working together – why close collaboration between continence and infection control services makes sense. *Continence*, **26** (3), 9.

Pratt, R.J., Pellowe, C.M., Wilson, J.A., Loveday, H.P., Jones, S.R., McDougall, C. and Wilcox, M.H. (2007) epic2: national evidence based guidelines for preventing healthcare associated infections in NHS hospitals in England. *Journal of Hospital Infection*, **65** (Suppl. 1, Feb.), S1–64.

Saint, S., Lipsky, B. and Goold, S.D. (2002) Indwelling urinary catheters: a one-point restraint? *Annals of Internal Medicine*, **137** (2), 125–127.

Saint, S., Kaufman, S.R., Thompson, M., Rogers, M.A.M. and Chenoweth, C. (2005) A reminder reduces urinary catheterisation in hospitalised patients. *Joint Commission Journal on Quality and Patient Safety*, **31** (8), 455–462.

Salgado, C.D., Karchmer, T.B. and Farr, B.M. (2003) Prevention of catheter associated urinary tract infections. In: *Prevention and Control of Nosocomial Infections* (ed. R.P. Wenzel) (fourth edition). Lippincott, Williams & Wilkins, Philadelphia.

Tambyah, P. (2004) Catheter associated urinary tract infections: diagnosis and prophylaxis *International Journal of Antimicrobial Agents*, **24S**, S44–88.

Tenke, P., Jackel, M. and Nagy, E. (2004) Prevention and treatment of catheter associated infections: myth or reality? *EUA Update Series*, **2**, 106–115.

Tew, L., Pomfret, I. and King, D. (2005) Infection risks associated with urinary catheters. *Nursing Standard*, **20** (7), 55–61.

Trauntner, B. and Darouiche, R. (2004) Role of biofilm in catheter associated urinary tract infection. *American Journal of Infection Control*, **32** (3), 177–183.

8 | Infection Prevention in Intravascular Therapy

Carly Hall

INTRODUCTION

Intravascular therapy is widely used in both acute and community healthcare settings. As well as delivering a range of intravenous (IV) fluids, including drugs, blood and blood products directly into the bloodstream, intravascular catheters can also be used to monitor acutely ill patients and to access blood samples. However, because of their invasive nature they can be an important cause of life threatening healthcare associated infection (HCAI).

The use of the word 'catheter' in this chapter refers to a flexible hollow tube, made from various materials including silicone, Teflon® and polyurethane that is introduced into the vascular system via veins and sometimes arteries. 'Cannula' is also used in the same sense. This chapter covers the principles of infection control relating to insertion and continuing care for a range of commonly used intravascular devices in adults.

LEARNING OBJECTIVES

By the end of the chapter you will be able to:

❏ Describe the infection risks associated with intravascular therapy, including routes of transmission and relevant micro-organisms
❏ Describe the infection prevention and control principles for insertion and management of key intravascular catheters and associated devices
❏ Describe the principles of line management and the optimum environment for preparing medication and equipment

INFECTION RISKS ASSOCIATED WITH INTRAVASCULAR THERAPY

Risks of infection for anyone receiving intravascular therapy can come from a number of different sources: from bacteria that live on the patient, which are referred to as normal flora – the exogenous route; and from micro-organisms that are found in the environment, which can be transferred to the patient – the endogenous route (Infection Control Nurses Association, 2001). If a person goes into hospital, is on long-term antibiotics, has an intravascular catheter inserted, or has a wound site, there is greater likelihood that their own micro-organisms and those from the environment may cause problems because the body's natural defences have been compromised.

Potential problems with any type of intravascular catheter include:

- Infection at the insertion site
- Infection where devices have been tunnelled through the skin
- Bloodstream infections (bacteraemias); a catheter related bloodstream infection (CR-BSI) is one where there is systemic infection and the catheter is the likely cause (Pratt *et al.*, 2007), for example if a patient develops an MRSA bacteraemia and is colonised with MRSA in their nose it is probable that there has been cross infection from nose to catheter site
- Endocarditis

THE MAIN WAYS MICRO-ORGANISMS ACCESS IV CATHETERS

Micro-organisms can reach catheter insertion sites in a number of ways: as a result of poor hand washing technique, lax practice around accessing intravascular devices and through contaminated equipment or fluids. Micro-organisms can then access intravascular catheters and enter the bloodstream by:

- **Externally migrating along the outside of the catheter from the insertion site**

This external route is associated with micro-organisms at the insertion site that may be the patient's normal skin flora or may have been transferred to the site from another source (e.g. hands of a healthcare worker or the patient themselves).

- **Entering the device and travelling along the inside lumen of the catheter**

This internal route is generally associated with bungs, three-way taps and other access points that are colonised, and fluids/drugs that may have been contaminated at the manufacturing, or at the preparation or drawing-up stage. If bungs, three-way taps and other access points are not adequately decontaminated, micro-organisms have the potential to enter cannulae. Three-way taps and extension lines can be problematic because if not flushed regularly organisms can grow in the small empty spaces (dead space) inside these devices and when a flush is given the patient is at risk of pathogenic micro-organisms directly entering the bloodstream.

- **Haematogenous spread**

Haematogenous spread involves micro-organisms from another area of the patient's body (e.g. from an infected or colonised wound site) migrating to the catheter site via the bloodstream. The catheter becomes colonised and can then potentially cause infection.

MICRO-ORGANISMS THAT CAN CAUSE INTRAVASCULAR DEVICE INFECTIONS

All micro-organisms have the potential to colonise catheter sites and go on to cause infection. *Staphylococci* spp. (bacteria), Gram negative rods (bacteria) and *Candida* spp. (fungi) are common organisms that can cause intravascular infections. *Staphylococcus epidermidis*, which is part of normal skin flora, can be problematic. This organism secretes a slime that helps it adhere to the outside of a catheter and migrate along it. *Staphylococcus aureus*, including meticillin resistant *Staphylococcus aureus* (MRSA), is often implicated; so too are the Gram negative organisms *Escherichia coli*, *Klebsiella* spp. and *Pseudomonas* spp.

KEY PRACTICES

Whatever the intravascular device, there are a number of key practices that significantly contribute to minimising the risks of infection.

Hand washing

If carrying out an aseptic technique (see below) hands should be cleansed with a preparation that is bactericidal (e.g. contains an active ingredient like chlorhexidine that kills most bacteria). Encourage patients to hand wash, especially after going to the toilet, because they could contaminate their own intravascular catheters and lines by touching them.

Aseptic technique

In relation to intravascular therapy 'aseptic technique' is a term that can be confusing and variously defined. The aim is to protect the patient from pathogenic micro-organisms accessing their intravascular device, the site around it and any drugs or fluids. Situations will differ so it is necessary to understand and apply the principles of asepsis. 'Aseptic non-touch technique' is a practical way of reducing risks to patients in situations involving intravascular devices. Used correctly it is possible to maintain asepsis by not touching 'key parts' of equipment that could become contaminated with micro-organisms and go on to contaminate the drugs or fluids entering the bloodstream (Rowley, 2001). However, there are instances when 'maximal sterile barrier precautions' are essential, for example during the insertion of a central line (Pratt *et al.*, 2007; Centers for Disease Control and Prevention, 2002; Pellowe *et al.*, 2004).

Selecting the right gloves

One area that can be unclear is which gloves should be worn for which practice. When caring for highly immune deficient patients, or carrying out lengthy or complex procedures, which involve line handling, giving drugs or inserting devices, then sterile gloves must be worn.

A skilled practitioner, who is able to avoid touching and contaminating key parts of a device or a skin area that has been decontaminated, may wear clean non-sterile latex (or nitrile) gloves; vinyl gloves are not advised.

Skin preparation

Various antiseptic solutions have been used over the years to render patient's skin as free from micro-organisms as possible prior to any invasive procedures. Currently, tincture of iodine, an iodophor or 70% alcohol can be used, but the recommended skin preparation solution in the USA is 2% chlorhexidine gluconate in 70% alcohol (Centers for Disease Control and Prevention, 2002). Pellowe *et al.* (2004) emphasise the need for this measure to be included in future UK guidelines for insertion and site care for all central venous catheters. This is being introduced into practice in the UK. Maki (2005) supports its use for all intravascular devices. However, the literature generally refers to using 70% alcohol for insertion of peripheral vascular catheters. It is the drying action of the alcohol that kills micro-organisms; therefore, alcohol must always be left to dry before commencing insertion. The benefit of chlorhexidine is that it will keep the area free from micro-organisms for a period of time even when the alcohol has dried.

Decontaminating access points
Bungs are the devices that seal and protect catheter lumens, lines and add-on devices. They can be simple bungs, injectable bungs, needle free connectors and valves or more complex implanted ports. They must always be decontaminated prior to being accessed. The same procedure must also be carried out if accessing other points in any IV system (e.g. three-way taps, access points in lines, access points in administration set burettes). A 70% alcohol wipe is usually sufficient, although some areas advocate wipes that contain 0.5% chlorhexidine gluconate in 70% alcohol. Rub the access point vigorously and allow to dry before accessing.

PERIPHERAL VENOUS CANNULAE (PVCS)

Insertion of PVCs
Prior to cannula insertion it is vital that an explanation of the procedure is given to the patient and that they understand what will happen, the risks involved and that they have given their consent (Dougherty and Lister, 2004; Royal College of Nursing, 2005). If the first attempt at cannulation is unsuccessful a new PVC must be used and the skin prepared again if the area has been palpated.

Equipment preparation

The equipment needed should be prepared before approaching the patient. Cannulation should be carried out using an aseptic technique. A plastic tray with an integral sharps bin should be used to carry items safely to the bedside and to dispose of sharps at the point of use. The smallest gauge cannulae required should be selected; the higher the number, the smaller the gauge (Royal College of Nursing, 2005). This helps minimise trauma to the vein which could contribute to infection (Infection Control Nurses Association, 2001). In emergencies larger gauge cannulae are often inserted in order to administer fluids quickly.

Selection of insertion site

Many factors need to be taken into consideration, including avoiding areas of flexion and the type of drugs to be given (Dougherty and Lister, 2004; Royal College of Nursing, 2005). The site selected may increase the risks of a catheter related infection; it is advisable to use the upper extremities as the risk of phlebitis is higher if the lower extremities are used (Infection Control Nurses Association, 2001; Centers for Disease Control and Prevention, 2002).

Patient's skin condition

Skin condition should be assessed prior to cannulation. In patients with skin conditions such as eczema or psoriasis it may be more difficult to prepare the skin adequately. Babies, young children and older people tend to have more fragile skin so take this into consideration particularly when removing cannula dressings.

Hand washing

Remove hand and wrist jewellery, including watches, and carry out a thorough systematic hand hygiene process before donning gloves pre-cannulation and post-cannulation after removing gloves (National Institute for Clinical Excellence, 2003).

Personal protective equipment (PPE)

Non-sterile latex or nitrile gloves can be used for peripheral cannulation. If there is a risk of being splashed by blood or body fluids, a disposable plastic apron and eye protection should be worn.

Skin preparation

Prepare the selected site vigorously with the chosen antiseptic. Use a circular movement, move away from the centre and allow the skin to dry.

Tourniquets

Single use disposable, latex-free tourniquets are advised to reduce risks of cross infection between patients. Fabric tourniquets are not advised as it is not possible to decontaminate them adequately between patients. Never use latex gloves as tourniquets. They are not designed for this and there are potential issues of latex allergy (Royal College of Nursing, 2005).

Dressing choice

A dressing for a peripheral cannula should be:

- Sterile
- Transparent
- Self-adhesive
- Semi-permeable
- Latex-free
- Easy to apply
- Easy to remove (Infection Control Nurses Association, 2001)

Apply the dressing as indicated by the manufacturer to ensure that the PVC remains stable and any movement in the vein is minimised. Many dressings include a small time and date label that can be secured on the dressing. The Infection Control Nurses Association (2006) advises that PVCs are labelled with an insertion date. Using the correct dressing obviates the need to bandage over the top. Bandages obscure sites and mean that they cannot be checked adequately.

Documentation

Cannula insertion and removal must be recorded in the patient's notes. Specifically record:

- Patient name/date of birth/hospital number/ward
- Cannula size

- Site inserted
- Inserted by
- Date and time inserted
- Dressing used
- VIP score sheet and record available
- Date cannula is removed
- Reason for removal
- Removed by
- Any problems
- Signature/job title of person carrying out procedures
- Contact number (Hyde, 2002; Royal College of Nursing, 2005; Infection Control Nurses Association, 2006)

Management of PVCs

• Checking the site; VIP scoring

The PVC site needs to be checked at least every shift. Some guidance indicates a minimum of once a day but problems can arise quickly. The device should be checked each time it is accessed. A visual inspection phlebitis score card – VIP (Jackson, 2003) can be used to assess the site.

• Initial signs of problems

Patient reports pain at the site or on use of device, redness near the site, erythema, swelling, VIP score 2 or above. If any of the above are apparent the PVC must be replaced and sited in a different place.

• Length of time a PVC should be in place

A patent cannula can stay in place for 72 hours and then it should be resited (DoH, 2005). If at 72 hours the device is not resited, the reasons must be clearly documented in the patient's notes. Always check the time and date label on the dressing/care plan. Cannulae sited in emergencies should be replaced within 24 hours (Royal College of Nursing, 2005).

• Checking the integrity of dressings

Quality sterile PVC dressings are designed to last longer than PVCs and should remain in place (72 hours). However, if there is excessive moisture build up, or the dressing becomes loose, it will need to be changed.

— Remove the dressing in the correct way to prevent minimal discomfort to the patient, movement of the PVC and trauma to the skin
— Use clean non-sterile latex or nitrile gloves
— Sterile gauze should be used to absorb any excess moisture
— Avoid touching the actual site with gloved hands
— Apply a new sterile dressing

- **Decontaminating bungs and access points**

Any access points should be decontaminated before and after using a 70% alcohol wipe, or an alcohol wipe containing chlorhexidine. Always allow to dry before accessing.

- **Removing cannulae**

PVCs should be removed as soon as they are no longer in use.

— Remove dressing and cover insertion site with sterile gauze
— Remove cannula gently and use sterile gauze to manage any bleeding
— Cover site with clean sterile gauze and tape until site has dried over

- **Documentation**

As with insertion, accurate documentation of PVC removal is important.

Complications with PVCs

- **Local problems**

Phlebitis is a general term for inflammation of the vein. This can occur for a number of reasons:

— *Mechanical phlebitis* can occur if the PVC is not securely fixed by a dressing. Movement of the catheter in the vein can result in trauma to the vein wall.
— *Chemical phlebitis* can occur as a result of some drugs, for example certain antibiotics and cytotoxic drugs, or a reaction to the cannula material.
— *Infection phlebitis* can occur as a result of micro-organisms causing an infection that affects the vein.

— *Thrombophlebitis* can occur when the vein has been inflamed or irritated in any way. A small blood clot can form which can lead to the vein becoming obstructed.

The symptoms of phlebitis are usually apparent; the site will feel tender to the patient and they may experience pain. It is likely that the site will look red and it may feel warm. Accessing the cannula with IV medication or fluids may be difficult and very uncomfortable for the patient. Other problems can occur with PVCs, including extravasation and infiltration; these are not specifically infection control problems but can compromise catheter sites in ways that can allow infection to develop more easily.

• **Systemic problems**
The major systemic problem related to all intravascular devices is bloodstream infection. All micro-organisms have the potential to cause CR-BSIs, which can be life threatening.

MIDLINE CATHETERS
Midline catheters are generally used for patients who need medium to long-term IV therapy (e.g. antibiotics, chemotherapy, pain management). They are inserted in large peripheral veins: basilic vein, median cubital vein or the cephalic vein, although the basilic is generally preferred. The length of the catheter inserted is usually between 7.5 and 20 cm and can be single or double lumen (Dougherty and Lister, 2004). Midline catheters do not extend beyond the axilla. This type of peripherally inserted catheter has benefits over short-term peripheral cannulae as it can stay in place longer, and also over central venous catheters in that potential complications of entering the central venous circulation are avoided.

Principles of insertion
Principles of insertion are similar to short-term PVCs. An aseptic technique should be used and the wearing of sterile gloves is advised (Dougherty and Lister, 2004). The actual insertion of midlines should only be carried out by staff trained in this procedure. Once inserted the device can be held in place by sterile adhesive tape, or a fixing device. A sterile, transparent,

semi-permeable dressing should be applied over the device, leaving the access port accessible.

Midline catheter management

- Always decontaminate bungs and access points before and after access.
- Dressings should be changed as stated in manufacturer's instructions, if they become loose or there is excessive moisture build up.
- For dressing changes use sterile gloves and cleanse the site with 2% chlorhexidine gluconate in 70% alcohol.
- Observe the site every shift and record the VIP score.

Removal of a midline

The literature is non-specific about how long a midline should remain in situ. The consensus is that they can stay in place for up to six weeks. If there are any signs of infection they must be removed.

- Remove the transparent dressing according to the manufacturer's instructions.
- Due to the fact that the midline can extend from 7.5 to 20 cm, care should be taken when removing the line to prevent trauma to the vein.
- Use sterile gauze to prevent bleeding and then cover the site with a small sterile dressing.
- Continue to observe the site to ensure that there are no localised problems.

Potential problems relating to midline catheters

Midlines are potentially able to cause the same local and systemic problems as short-term cannulae. Jones (2004) indicates that phlebitis is less of a problem in midlines than short-term PVCs. However, it is still vital to observe the site regularly, use the VIP scoring chart and document the findings.

PERIPHERAL ARTERIAL CATHETERS

Peripheral arterial catheters are generally used for continuous monitoring of inter-arterial blood pressure in critically ill patients.

They also facilitate easy access for taking blood samples. The most common insertion site is the radial artery, but other sites include the femoral and axillary arteries (Scheer *et al.*, 2002).

Principles of insertion

- Prepare all equipment in a clean environment.
- Someone trained in the procedure should perform the actual insertion.
- Particular attention should be paid to pre-insertion hand washing and skin preparation of the patient.
- An aseptic technique should be used and sterile gloves worn.
- A sterile, transparent, semi-permeable dressing should be applied over the device.

Management of peripheral arterial catheters

Peripheral arterial catheter sites need to be observed every shift and this should be documented. If there are any signs of infection or the patient is experiencing pain report this to the medical staff. To keep arterial lines patent an infusion is set up under pressure so that the line can be flushed easily. In order to manage this infusion and access the line for blood samples a three-way tap is commonly used. Prior to starting any procedure with a peripheral arterial catheter, hands should be decontaminated and gloves worn.

When taking a blood sample ensure that before the cap on the three-way tap is removed the port is decontaminated. If there is a different access system in place it should also be decontaminated. The port/access point should also be decontaminated when the procedure is finished. If the port is capped with a simple bung a new sterile bung should be used after every access. Disposable or reusable transducers attached to the peripheral arterial catheter system should be replaced every 96 hours. Guidelines advise that all other components of the system should be changed at the same intervals (Centers for Disease Control and Prevention, 2002). Thorough aseptic technique and appropriate cleaning of the insertion site are important factors in helping to decrease the likelihood of a catheter related infection (Scheer *et al.*, 2002).

Removal of a peripheral arterial catheter

- Prepare the equipment, decontaminate hands and don gloves.
- Remove the dressing.
- Clean around the site with 2% chlorhexidine gluconate in 70% alcohol.
- Pressure will need to be applied to the site after catheter removal prior to covering with a small sterile dressing.
- Observe the site for a short time after to ensure no complications occur.

Potential problems relating to peripheral arterial catheters

Problems with peripheral arterial catheters usually relate to temporary occlusion of the artery. It would appear that a major risk of infection and sepsis is related to the time the catheter is in situ. Problems tend to arise when they have been in situ longer than 96 hours. Evidence indicates that the rate of CR-BSI in peripheral arterial catheters is comparable to those in short-term CVCs (Centers for Disease Control and Prevention, 2002).

CENTRAL VENOUS CATHETERS (CVCS)

CVCs are used for the administration of drugs and fluids, total parenteral nutrition (TPN) and also for haemodynamic monitoring. The nature of CVCs means that they are suitable for infusing large volumes of IV fluid and blood, and can deliver drugs that may irritate small peripheral veins. It is advised that 'the minimum number of ports and lumens essential for the management of the patient' are used (Centers for Disease Control and Prevention, 2002).

CVCs are often inserted via the subclavian, jugular or femoral veins and catheter tips normally sit in the superior vena cava, inferior vena cava or right atrium (Dougherty, 2000). There is some evidence that subclavian insertion causes fewer problems with infection (Infection Control Nurses Association, 2001). If there is a need for hair removal this should be carried out with clippers rather than a razor to prevent small cuts and abrasions that could contribute to infection.

CVCs can also be inserted by the peripheral routes using the basilic, cephalic or brachial veins. These are known as PICC (peripherally inserted central catheter) lines (Jones, 2004) and will be discussed shortly.

Apart from PICCs the main types of CVC that you will come across are:

- **Short-term, non-tunnelled CVCs**
These are designed to be used for up to a few weeks. They are sutured in place at the insertion site, or secured with a fixing device, and should be covered with a sterile, transparent, semipermeable dressing (National Institute for Clinical Excellence, 2003; Infection Control Nurses Association, 2006). This type of CVC accounts for a significant number of CR-BSI (Pratt *et al.*, 2007; Centers for Disease Control and Prevention, 2002).

- **Long-term, skin tunnelled CVCs**
Pratt *et al.* (2007) advise that if patients are expected to need vascular access for longer than 30 days then they should have a tunnelled catheter or implantable access device. These types of CVC can stay in place for many months. They are tunnelled under the skin and have a cuff that 'bonds' with the surrounding tissue to help secure it in place. They are frequently used for administration of chemotherapy and TPN. They tend to have a lower rate of CR-BSI because the cuff helps stop micro-organisms migrating along the outside of the lumen.

Principles of insertion
All short-term, non-tunnelled and long-term tunnelled CVCs should be inserted using maximal sterile barrier precautions by medical staff that are trained in the procedure (Pratt *et al.*, 2007; Centers for Disease Control and Prevention, 2002).

Management of CVCs
Skilled management of all CVCs is essential to minimise the risks of infection and you should check local guidelines/policies for recommended practice in your area. However, as with all intravascular lines similar basic principles are relevant.

- **Accessing lines/add-on devices**
  - Do not access lines unless essential
  - Decontaminate hands before donning and after removing gloves
  - Assess the need for the use of sterile or non-sterile gloves
  - Assess the need for other personal protective equipment
  - Decontaminate any hubs/bungs/add-on devices before and after accessing
  - Always make sure each lumen of the CVC is sealed with a bung

If TPN is being given an individual CVC should be used or one lumen dedicated for this (Pratt *et al.*, 2007).

- **Dressings and CVCs**

Either sterile gauze or sterile, transparent, semi-permeable dressings can be used to cover the CVC site (Centers for Disease Control and Prevention, 2002). In practice the latter is advised on short-term, non-tunnelled CVCs because these dressings are designed to stay in place longer, are more secure and the site can be observed. Transparent dressings should be changed every seven days or sooner if loose, or they have excessive moisture build up. Once a long-term, tunnelled CVC insertion site is healed it no longer needs a dressing. Changing dressings requires an aseptic technique using sterile gloves. Clean the exit site with 2% chlorhexidine gluconate in 70% alcohol, allow to dry and then apply a new sterile dressing.

- **Observation of site and documentation**

The CVC site should be observed every time it is accessed, or at least every shift. If the patient shows local or systemic signs of infection report this immediately as the device may need to be removed. Good documentation around all aspects of CVC care is critical.

Removal of CVCs

Care needs to be taken to prevent the site becoming contaminated in any way. Once the suture or fixing device is removed, place sterile gauze over the CVC and remove the CVC following the recommended procedure. When any bleeding has stopped cover the site with a small sterile transparent dressing. Observe over a few days to ensure there are no localised problems.

Potential problems relating to CVCs

The main problem relating to CVCs are bloodstream infections. These infections can be life threatening and require careful management and often IV antibiotics.

PERIPHERALLY INSERTED CENTRAL VENOUS CATHETERS (PICCS)

As with midlines, PICCs are generally used for patients who need medium to long-term IV therapy (e.g. antibiotics and chemotherapy). However, whilst PICCs are inserted peripherally they are positioned in the superior vena cava (Dougherty, 2000). Similar veins are used to midline insertion. The length of the catheter inserted is usually between 50–70 cm and can be single or double lumen (Philpot and Griffiths, 2003). These catheters have advantages over PVCs and midlines in that they deliver drugs and fluids centrally, but few of the disadvantages of short-term CVCs; exit sites in awkward areas can be hard to manage and more prone to microbial contamination.

Principles of insertion

Increasingly, nurses who have been specially trained in this procedure are inserting PICCs.

- An aseptic technique should be used for insertion, including sterile gloves (Philpot and Griffiths, 2003).

- Once the PICC is in situ, a sterile, transparent, semi-permeable dressing should be applied at the exit site. There may be some bleeding in the first 24 hours so this first dressing may require a small square of sterile gauze under the transparent dressing. After 24 hours this can be carefully removed and replaced with a new sterile transparent dressing (no gauze).

- PICCs need to be secured to the skin so that the catheter does not move. Different techniques can be used: suturing, tape or a fixing device. Whatever is used should be sterile and allow observation of the site.

Management of PICCs

- Access valves, connectors and hubs should be decontaminated before and after they are accessed.
- Use an aseptic technique with sterile gloves for dressing changes.
- Clean the exit site with 2% chlorhexidine gluconate in 70% alcohol, allow to dry then apply a new sterile dressing.
- The site should be observed every shift when first inserted and then once daily and the VIP score recorded on the appropriate documentation.

Removal of a PICC

General guidelines do not state how long a PICC can remain in place (Infection Control Nurses Association, 2001). If there are any signs of infection the PICC must be removed.

- Care should be taken to prevent the site becoming contaminated.
- An aseptic technique should be used.
- Remove the dressing and fixing device.
- Place sterile gauze over the PICC and remove following the recommended procedure.
- When any bleeding has stopped cover the site with a small, sterile, transparent dressing that should stay in place for 72 hours.
- Observe for any localised problems.

Potential infection control problems relating to PICCs

The various types of phlebitis discussed earlier can potentially cause problems for patients with PICCs. However, PICCs tend to be associated with lower rates of CR-BSI.

IMPLANTED VENOUS ACCESS PORTS

Implanted venous access ports are used when patients need long-term vascular access in hospital and the community (e.g. for long-term antibiotics or chemotherapy). A catheter is centrally inserted and then connected to a port that has been surgically placed in a pocket under the skin. Ports come in different sizes and are made from various materials. They are generally sited in the arm or upper chest wall area. Implantable port insertion is a surgical procedure that takes place under general or local anaesthetic.

Management of implantable ports
Once the skin has healed over the port, risks of infection are minimal. Ports can be used to take blood, give bolus drugs or for administration of medication over a longer period.

- An aseptic technique should be used and sterile gloves worn.
- The skin around and over the port should be decontaminated prior to access.
- If patients need local anaesthetic on the port site to minimise pain from needle insertion this can be applied after skin/port preparation but must be sterile and from a single use applicator.
- For medication administration over a number of days a non-coring needle is passed through the self-sealing septum of the port which has been designed to be accessed many times (around 2000 punctures). The needle sits in the chamber of the port and medication passes through this into the venous system.
- Whilst the port needle is in situ it needs to be supported with sterile gauze and covered with a sterile transparent dressing so that the needle stays in the port (Dougherty and Lister, 2004). If it moves extravasation can take place.

Potential problems relating to implantable ports
Although risks of infection are reduced with ports, the site should be observed regularly and the patient encouraged to report any signs of infection. As with insertion, port removal is a surgical procedure.

ASSOCIATED INTRAVASCULAR CATHETER DEVICES
There are a number of devices that can be added to catheters either directly or via lines. Every effort should be made to reduce the number of lines, lumens and stopcocks to a minimum (DoH, 2003). Where vascular add-on devices are used they must be

changed at least as frequently as when the catheter or administration set is changed or if the integrity of either product is compromised (Registered Nurses' Association of Ontario, 2005).

Stopcocks (three-way taps/extension sets) must always be flushed thoroughly and capped after each use. If contaminated with blood products, lipid emulsions or drugs, they should be replaced. Whenever a cap is removed from the circuit, it should be replaced with a sterile one (Infection Control Nurses Association, 2001). Needle-free connectors are beneficial in maintaining closed systems and potentially reducing sharps injuries. Education and training around their use must be provided and the connectors should be decontaminated before and after being accessed. They are generally designed to be used for a specific number of activations or days, whichever comes sooner. There is no definitive evidence to suggest that in-line filters are effective in preventing CR-BSIs associated with intravascular catheters and infusion systems (Centers for Disease Control and Prevention, 2002).

Principles of line management

Administration sets (giving sets) are the lines that attach to catheters and deliver fluids and drugs. They can attach directly to catheter hubs or via other routes such as a three-way tap. Administration sets should be changed at regular intervals. Table 8.1 details the recommended change times.

Changing fluid bags

If a patient is having, for example, two (litre) bags of sodium chloride 0.9% over 24 hours, one administration set can be used. Care should be taken when changing the bags. Hands should be washed and the spike on the administration set should not be touched.

Labelling of administration sets/and fluids

Administration sets for all fluids and medication, and bags of fluid should be labelled with the date/time they are prepared for use and the fluid/medication that is going through the set. If patients have more than one line, they must be marked (e.g. A, B, C) so that lumens are dedicated.

Table 8.1 Recommended times for changing intravascular administration sets (Infection Control Nurses Association, 2001; Centers for Disease Control and Prevention, 2002; National Institute for Clinical Excellence, 2003; Registered Nurses' Association of Ontario, 2005; Pratt *et al.*, 2007).

Solution type	Administration set change
Sodium chloride 0.9%	At 72 hours or immediately if any problems become apparent
Lipids	At 24 hours or immediately if any problems become apparent
Whole blood	At least every 12 hours for a continuing transfusion and when the transfusion has been completed
Platelets	Once infusion is completed the set must be discarded and not used for any other solution
Intermittent infusions, for example IV antibiotics	If set is disconnected from the patient it should be discarded immediately If set remains connected to the patient the set should stay in situ for 24 hours Change immediately any problems become apparent

Principles of drug and equipment preparation

- There should be a designated area where medication and fluids are prepared.
- Ensure any surfaces have been decontaminated and are dry before commencing preparation.
- Principles of asepsis should be adhered to.
- Hands must be decontaminated prior to commencing preparation.
- Risk assess the need for wearing gloves – generally it will be sufficient to wear non-sterile gloves as long as key parts of the equipment are not touched.
- If drawing up sodium chloride/sterile water from small plastic ampoules (5/10 ml) it is important to use a needle. Do not break the ampoule tops and insert a syringe directly into the ampoule. Needle tips are sterile but the outside of plastic vials are not and there is potential for the flush to become contaminated.

- If drawing up antibiotics in syringes for bolus use protect the syringe tip by leaving needles on syringes until the point of administration.
- Avoid multi-dose vials. Decontaminate the bungs of vials with an alcohol wipe before accessing.
- Use a plastic tray with an integral sharps bin to take any IV drugs/subcutaneous drugs to the bedside. Discard sharps at the point of use.
- Do not touch the spike of any administration set.
- Once bag seal and tag have been broken take care to avoid contamination of the spike during insertion.
- Ensure a sterile bung is placed on the end of the administration set if the fluids are being prepared prior to going to a patient.

EXERCISE

Jackson (2003) lists 28 potential problems that can arise with intravascular therapy and access but indicates that this is probably not exhaustive. Make a two-column table. On the left-hand side write down as many problems as you can relating to intravascular devices and issues that could arise as a result of poor infection control practice. On the right-hand side, against each problem, write down how these problems could be prevented.

SUMMARY

Intravascular therapy places patients at risk of local infection from the catheter insertion site and life threatening bloodstream infection. Infection prevention practices comprise good aseptic technique for insertion and all handling, as well as regular observation and documentation of the catheter site.

REFERENCES

Centers for Disease Control and Prevention (2002) Guidelines for the prevention of intravascular catheter related infections. *Morbidity and Mortality Weekly Review*, **51**, RR–10.
Department of Health (2003) *Winning Ways. Working Together to Reduce Healthcare Associated Infection in England*. Department of Health, London.

Department of Health (2005) *Saving Lives: a Delivery Programme to Reduce Healthcare Associated Infection Including MRSA*. Department of Health, London.

Dougherty, L. (2000) Central venous access devices. *Nursing Standard*, **14** (43), 45–50.

Dougherty, L. and Lister, S. (eds) (2004) *The Royal Marsden Hospital Manual of Clinical Nursing Procedures* (sixth edition). Blackwell Publishing, Oxford.

Hyde, L. (2002) Legal and professional aspects of intravenous therapy. *Nursing Standard*, **16** (26), 39–42.

Infection Control Nurses Association (2001) *Guidelines for Preventing Intravascular Catheter-related Infection*. Infection Control Nurses Association, Bathgate.

Infection Control Nurses Association (2006) *PIVA: Preventing Infections in Vascular Access Toolkit*. Infection Control Nurses Association, Bathgate.

Jackson, A. (2003) Reflecting on the nursing contribution to vascular access. *British Journal of Nursing*, **12** (11), 657–665.

Jones, A. (2004) Dressings for the management of catheter sites. *Journal of the Association of Vascular Access*, **9** (1), 26–33.

Maki, D. (2005) Renowned expert Dennis Maki, MD, addresses catheter related infections. *Infection Control Today*, **9** (1). Available at: www.infectioncontroltoday.com/articles/511fcat3.html (accessed 15 November 2006).

National Institute for Clinical Excellence (2003) *Infection Control. Prevention of Healthcare Associated Infection in Primary and Community Care*. Clinical Guideline 2. NICE, London.

Pellowe, C.M., Pratt, R.J., Loveday, H.P., Harper, P., Robinson, N. and Jones, S.R.L.J. (2004) The *epic* project. Updating the evidence base for national evidence based guidelines for preventing healthcare associated infections in NHS hospitals in England: a report with recommendations. *British Journal of Infection Control*, **5** (6), 10–16.

Philpot, P. and Griffiths, V. (2003) The peripherally inserted central catheter. *Nursing Standard*, **17** (44), 39–46.

Pratt, R.J., Pellowe, C.M., Wilson, J.A., Loveday, H.P., Jones, S.R., McDougall, C. and Wilcox, M.H. (2007) epic2: national evidence based guidelines for preventing healthcare associated infections in NHS hospitals in England. *Journal of Hospital Infection*, **65** (Suppl. 1, Feb.), S1–64.

Registered Nurses' Association of Ontario (2005) *Care and Maintenance to Reduce Vascular Access Complications. Nursing Best Practice Guideline*. Registered Nurses' Association of Ontario, Ontario.

Rowley, S. (2001) Aseptic non-touch technique. *NT Plus*, **97** (7), vi–viii.

Royal College of Nursing IV Therapy Forum (2005) *Standards for Infusion Therapy*. Royal College of Nursing, London.

Scheer, B.V., Perel, A. and Pfeiffer, U.J. (2002) Clinical review: complications and risk factors of peripheral arterial catheters used for haemodynamic monitoring in anaesthesia and intensive care medicine. *Critical Care*, **6** (3), 199–204.

Infection Prevention in Nutritional Care

9

INTRODUCTION

Adequate nutrition is important in a hospital to maintain a patient's immune function, healing capacity and general strength. Where patients are unable to obtain nutrition through normal dietary means, feeding by the enteral and parenteral route is often used. Enteral feeding places patients at increased risk of infection due to the invasive nature of tubes used to administer the feed and through the risk of contamination of the feeding solutions. Patients receiving parenteral feeding are at even greater risk of infection due to the direct access of the intravenous line into the bloodstream and the microbial growth supporting characteristics of intravenous feeding solutions.

LEARNING OBJECTIVES

By the end of this chapter you will be able to:

❏ Discuss the micro-organisms associated with infection in enteral and parenteral feeding
❏ Identify routes and points of entry for potential contamination
❏ Describe infection prevention measures for enteral and parenteral feeding

ENTERAL FEEDING

Enteral feeding is used in hospitals to ensure patients receive adequate nutrition if they are not able to take food and fluid through the conventional route. Inadequate nutrition in hospital can lead to patients having a lowered immunity to infection, poor wound healing and poor muscle strength, with undernourished patients staying in hospital an average of five additional days

(Stroud *et al.*, 2003). Enteral nutrition can be administered by a number of routes:

- Nasogastric
- Nasojejunal
- Percutaneous gastrostomy
- Percutaneous gastrojejunostomy
- Percutaneous jejunostomy

Although enteral feeding places patients at risk of infection, this is less than the infection risk associated with parenteral nutrition via the intravascular route and is, therefore, the preferred route for feeding, providing the patient does not have any mechanical complications affecting absorption of feed.

Infection associated with enteral feeding is not restricted to gastro-intestinal disease; sepsis, pneumonia and urinary tract infections have been associated with enteral feeding (Stroud *et al.*, 2003). Micro-organisms that have been reported as associated with contamination of enteral feed include:

- *Salmonella*
- *Enterococcus* spp.
- Coliforms (Oliviera *et al.*, 2000)

Contamination can be introduced into an enteral feeding system at a number of points and by a variety of routes:

- Touch contamination of equipment used for preparing and administering the feed
- Storage of prepared feeds in a contaminated area
- Failure to store feeds under refrigerated conditions where required
- Contamination of opened feed that has not been discarded when required
- Contamination of feeds during preparation
- Use of contaminated feeding ingredients
- Reuse and inadequate decontamination of equipment used for preparation and administration of feed
- Reuse or topping up of feed containers

- Connections within the system, for example drug administration/flushing port
- Introduction of micro-organisms from the nose and nasal pharynx on insertion
- Overgrowth of bacteria on the surfaces of the feeding tube (Anderton, 1995; Skipper *et al.*, 2003)

The following principles should be applied to the management of all enteral feeding, regardless of route (American Gastoenterological Association, 1995; Medical Devices Agency, 2000; National Institute for Clinical Excellence, 2003; Skipper *et al.*, 2003; Stroud *et al.*, 2003).

Equipment

- Feed containers should have lids that can be easily removed without risk of contamination.
- Pumps should be easily cleanable, with flush touch panels as opposed to grooves and buttons, wherever possible.
- An administration system that minimises the number of connections and access points should be used in preference.
- Extension tubes and three-way taps should be avoided.
- Feeding system components that are designated as single use should not be reprocessed or reused.
- Dislodged feeding tubes that are classified as single use should not be re-passed.
- Reusable equipment must be processed in accordance with the manufacturer's instructions.
- Bottle openers should be dedicated to enteral feeding use and should be disinfected with an alcohol wipe before use.
- Scissors used for contact with the feeding equipment should be sterile at the point of use.
- Sterile, ready to administer feeds should be used in preference to those that have to be reconstituted or decanted.

Storage of feed

- Ready to use feed should be stored in a clean environment and should be protected from extremes of temperature.

- Stock should be rotated to ensure feed is used within the expiry date.
- Reconstituted and opened feeds that are not being immediately administered should be refrigerated and used within 24 hours.
- Feeds that require refrigeration should be stored in a dedicated refrigerator and should not be stored with drugs or specimens.
- The refrigerator temperature should be between 1–4°C. The temperature should be monitored and recorded twice daily.
- The time and date of reconstitution or opening should be clearly labelled on stored feed.

Feed preparation

- Feed preparation should be carried out with the same principles applied to general food handling; in particular, staff with skin or wound infections, sore throats, diarrhoea and/or vomiting should not be involved in feed preparation or administration.
- Staff should be adequately trained in food hygiene and enteral feed preparation techniques.
- When reconstituting or decanting feeds this should be done in a clean environment.
- The working surface for feed preparation should be clean before the procedure commences.
- An aseptic technique should be used for all feed preparation, paying particular attention to hand hygiene.
- Sterile water should be used for feed reconstitution for all hospital in-patients.
- Gloves and aprons may be worn in accordance with hospital policy.

Feed administration

- An aseptic technique should be used for feed administration, paying particular attention to hand hygiene.
- Continuous feeding may lead to a rise in gastric pH, supporting bacterial overgrowth. Bolus feeding or intermittent feeding

may reduce gastric colonisation levels (Skiest and Metersky, 1997).

- Patients who are at risk of aspiration, which could lead to pneumonia, should not be fed at night if possible.
- Staff administering feed should be adequately trained in food hygiene and administration techniques.
- Ready to use sterile feeds should be used wherever possible.
- Sterile feeds should not be decanted for administration unless absolutely necessary, for example the volume of feed is too great for total administration.
- If decanting feed, the top of the feed container and the feed reservoir should be disinfected with alcohol and allowed to dry.
- Protective clothing should be worn in accordance with hospital policy.
- An aseptic non-touch technique (see Chapter 8) should be used for connecting the administration set to the feeding tube, taking care not to cause contamination by touching patient clothing.
- Ready prepared sterile feeds should be discarded after hanging for a maximum of 24 hours. If the feed is disconnected, the disconnection time is counted within the 24 hours.
- Sterile feeds that have been decanted into a sterile reservoir aseptically should be discarded after hanging for a maximum of 24 hours.
- Reconstituted feed and non-sterile feeds should be discarded after hanging for a maximum of four hours.
- Administration sets that are single use should be used out of preference in hospital settings and should be discarded after each feeding session.
- The administration set should not be disconnected during a feeding session unless essential. Administration of medications should be undertaken through a drug/flushing port to avoid disconnection.
- Following feed and drug administration, the feeding tube should be flushed with 30 mls of sterile water to remove deposits that might support microbial growth. A large volume syringe should be used to reduce the risk of feeding tube rupture.

INSERTION AND CARE OF NASALLY
INSERTED FEEDING TUBES

Nasogastric and nasojejunal tubes are inserted via the nasal passages into the gastro-intestinal system. It is common for these types of tubes to be inserted in the ward or department setting as opposed to an operating room environment. They are generally used when the period for feeding is likely to be less than six weeks. Fine bore polyurethane or silicone tubes should be used in preference to large bore PVC tubes, which may lead to increased gastric reflux and aspiration as well as causing damage to the nose and oesophagus (Stroud *et al.*, 2003). The tube should be inserted using an aseptic technique. Care should be taken not to contaminate the tube before insertion into the patient's nasal passage. For ongoing care and management, an aseptic technique should be used for all handling of the tube. Protective clothing should be worn, based on a risk assessment of the likely contact with gastric fluid. Where the tip of the feeding tube lies past the pylorus there is a greater risk of infective complications as the effect of the low gastric pH in reducing infection risk is not present; sterile water should always be used for post-pyloric feeding and flushing.

INSERTION AND MANAGEMENT OF PERCUTANEOUSLY
INSERTED FEEDING TUBES

In addition to infection risks associated with the administration of a food substance, percutaneously inserted feeding tubes have the risk of exit site and peritoneal infection. Percutaneous feeding tubes (PETs) are inserted surgically through a stoma in the abdominal wall into the stomach (percutaneous endoscopic gastrostomy) or into the jejunum (percutaneous endoscopic jejunostomy). Exit site infections in PETs may be as high as 15% (Löser *et al.*, 2005) and are generally noted in the immediate time period after insertion of the tube (National Institute for Clinical Excellence, 2003). Micro-organisms that can cause exit site infection are those most associated with wound infection and include *Staphylococcus aureus* (including meticillin resistant – MRSA), *Streptococcus pyogenes* and pseudomonads (Chaudhary *et al.*, 2004). Exit site infection is characterised by redness around the stoma, pain, pus production and fever. Slight redness (up to 5 mm) is common after PET insertion and may not be an indication of infection. To reduce the risk of exit site infection, antibiotic prophylaxis can be given at the time of PET insertion (Lipp and Lusardi, 2006). Once the exit site stoma has healed it can be washed daily with soap and water and dried (National Institute for Clinical Excellence, 2003). Prior to this time, an aseptic technique and disinfection of the exit site should be performed and a sterile dressing applied (Löser *et al.*, 2005).

Procedure for daily dressing of PET exit site until stoma healed

The dressing procedure should be carried out using the principles of asepsis described in Chapter 10:

- Explain the procedure to the patient and obtain their consent to perform the procedure.
- Prepare equipment required, including dressing trolley and sterile dressing pack.
- Decontaminate hands and prepare sterile dressing field.
- Wearing non-sterile gloves, remove the old dressing and discard as clinical waste.
- Remove gloves, discard as clinical waste and decontaminate hands (alcohol hand gel is useful in these circumstances as it can be applied at the bedside).
- Don sterile gloves and clean the exit site with sterile saline if there is any exudate present.
- Disinfect the exit site using a circular motion moving in concentric circles away from the stoma.
- Apply the sterile dressing.
- Dispose of the dressing equipment and make the patient comfortable.
- Record the dressing procedure and the appearance of the stoma site in the patient's record.

For gastrostomy tubes only, the tube is rotated to avoid adhesions and buried bumper syndrome, which is where the gastric mucosa partly or fully grows over the internal bolster of the tube (National Institute for Clinical Excellence, 2003; Löser *et al.*, 2005).

PARENTERAL FEEDING

Parenteral nutrition (PN) is used to provide nutrition to patients who do not have an adequately functioning gut, for example patients with short bowel syndrome, malabsorption syndromes or prolonged paralytic ileus. It involves the direct infusion of essential nutrients into a vein (Dougherty and Lister, 2004). Infusion is generally via a catheter inserted into a central vein; however, PN can be administered into a peripherally inserted central venous catheter if given with care. Catheter related infection is probably the complication of most concern associated with parenteral nutrition (Deshpande, 2003). Higher rates of catheter associated infection have been reported when PN is being administered as opposed to other solutions (Richet *et al.*, 1990; Moro *et al.*, 1994). However, more recently it has been suggested that rates of infection can be lowered to be comparable or less than those reported for central venous catheters by adhering to good principles of infection prevention (Dimick *et al.*, 2003). Outbreaks of infection have also been associated with contamination of PN solutions (Tresoldi *et al.*, 2000). Intravascular catheters used for administration of PN should be cared for in accordance with the principles of care described in Chapter 8. These following additional principles should be applied to care of PN catheters:

- An aseptic non-touch technique must be used for all handling of the PN line and directly associated equipment.
- Staff must be competent in aseptic non-touch technique before handling PN lines and carrying out dressing changes.
- A single lumen line dedicated to PN use should be used out of preference.
- Three-way taps and ports should not be added to the line.
- Unnecessary handling of the line must be avoided.
- The PN line must only be used for the administration of other solutions and drugs in exceptional circumstances.
- The infusion line must be changed every 24 hours if a lipid solution is being infused. (Centers for Disease Prevention and Control, 2002; Dimick *et al.*, 2003; Essex Critical Care Network, 2003).

SCENARIO

Mr Parry is a 68-year-old man who has had a percutaneous endo-scopic gastrostomy tube (PET) inserted due to swallowing difficulties following a cerebrovascular accident. What are the immediate care management requirements to prevent infection?

In the immediate post-operative period the PET should be handled with an aseptic technique for dressing changes. A sterile dressing should be applied. The stoma should be checked at each dressing change for signs of infection, including redness, pain and purulent exudate. The tube should be gently rotated to prevent buried bumper syndrome.

SUMMARY

Patients receiving enteral and parenteral nutrition are at increased risk of infection due to the presence of invasive devices. Risk of infection is also increased as the nutrient solutions provide an ideal environment to support microbial growth. Feeding by the enteral route reduces the risk of serious infection, but whichever route is used, good infection control practice is required at all times.

REFERENCES

American Gastroenterological Association (1995) *Medical Position Statement: Guidelines for Use of Enteral Nutrition*. American Gastro-enterological Association, Bethesda.

Anderton, A. (1995) Reducing bacterial contamination in enteral tube feeds. *British Journal of Nursing*, **4** (7), 368–376.

Centers for Disease Control and Prevention (2002) Guidelines for the prevention of intravascular catheter related infections. *Morbidity and Mortality Weekly Review*, **51**, RR–10.

Chaudhary, K.A., Smith, O.J., Cuddy, P.G. and Clarkston, W.K. (2004) PEG site infections: the emergence of meticillin resistant *Staphylococcus aureus* as a major pathogen. *American Journal of Gastroenterology*, **97** (7), 1713–1716.

Deshpande, K. (2003) Total parenteral nutrition and infections associated with use of central venous catheters. *American Journal of Critical Care*, **12** (4), 326–380.

Dimick, J.B., Swoboda, S., Talamini, M.A., Pelz, R.K., Hendrix, C.W. and Lipsett, P.A. (2003) Risk of colonisation of central venous catheters: catheters for total parenteral nutrition vs other catheters. *American Journal of Critical Care*, **12** (4), 328–335.

Dougherty, L. and Lister, S. (eds) (2004) *The Royal Marsden Hospital Manual of Clinical Nursing Procedures* (sixth edition). Blackwell Publishing, Oxford.

Essex Critical Care Network (2003) *TPN Care Bundle* Available at: http://www.sussexcritcare.nhs.uk/profclinical/carebundles/documents/TPNcarebundleguidelines.pdf (accessed 1 April 2006).

Lipp, A. and Lusardi, G. (2006) Systematic antimicrobial prophylaxis for percutaneous endoscopic gastrostomy. *Cochrane Database of Systemic Reviews*, **4**, Art. No. CD005571.

Löser, Chr., Aschl, G., Hébuterne, X. *et al.* (2005) ESPEN guidelines on artificial enteral nutrition – percutaneous endoscopic gastrostomy (PEG). *Clinical Nutrition*, **24**, 848–861.

Medical Devices Agency (2000) Safety Notice SN 2000 (27) *Enteral Feeding Systems*. Medical Devices Agency, London.

Moro, M.L., Vigano, E.F. and Cossi Lepri, A. (1994) Risk factors for central venous catheter related infections in surgical and intensive care units. *Infection Control Hospital Epidemiology*, **15** (4), 253–264.

National Institute for Clinical Excellence (2003) *Prevention of Healthcare Associated Infections in Primary and Community Care. Section 4 – Enteral Feeding*. National Institute for Clinical Excellence, London.

Oliviera, M.H., Bonelli, R., Aidoo, K.E. and Batista, C.R. (2000) Microbiological quality of reconstituted enteral formulations used in hospitals. *Nutrition*, **16** (9), 729–733.

Richet, H., Hubert, B., Nitemberg, F.Y. *et al.* (1990) Prospective multicenter study of vascular-catheter-related complications and risk factors for positive central-catheter cultures in intensive care unit patients. *Journal of Clinical Microbiology*, **28**, 2520–2525.

Skiest, D.J. and Metersky, M.L. (1997) The role of intermittent enteral feeding in reducing gastric colonisation in mechanically ventilated patients. *Chest*, **111** (5), 1474–1475.

Skipper, L., Cuffling, J. and Pratelli, N. (2003) *Enteral Feeding: Infection Control Guidelines*. Infection Control Nurses Association, Edinburgh.

Stroud, M., Duncan, H. and Nightingale, J. (2003) Guidelines for enteral feeding in hospital patients. *Gut*, **52** (suppl. VII), vii1–12.

Tresoldi, A.T., Padoveze, M.C., Trabasso, P. *et al.* (2000) *Enterobacter cloacae* sepsis outbreak in a newborn unit caused by contaminated total parenteral nutrition solution. *American Journal of Infection Control*, **28** (3), 258–261.

Infection Prevention in Wound Management

10

INTRODUCTION

Any wound, whether acute or chronic, places patients at risk of infection due to the breach in the body's defence from an intact skin. Chronic wounds are often colonised with bacteria, which could progress to cause infection. Within the hospital setting wounds should be managed using techniques that help prevent endogenous and exogenous infection. This chapter covers infection prevention during management of acute and chronic wounds.

LEARNING OBJECTIVES

By the end of this chapter you will be able to:

❏ Identify bacteria that are likely to cause infection in acute wounds and those that may be colonising chronic wounds
❏ Describe the principles of performing an aseptic and a clean technique
❏ Discuss the management of infected wounds

THE NATURE OF WOUNDS

Wounds can be classified into acute wounds and chronic wounds. Acute wounds usually heal within four weeks and follow the normal phases of healing; chronic wounds generally do not heal within four weeks and appear not to follow the normal process of wound healing (McGuckin *et al.*, 2003). Wound healing occurs in a continuous manner, but different phases are often seen in the process:

• The inflammatory response – erythema, swelling, heat and pain
• Collagen synthesis – tissue regeneration

- Angiogenesis – new blood vessel formation
- Epithelialisation – regrowth of skin
- Maturation – strengthening of new tissue (Gould, 2001)

Acute wounds that follow the processes above are also sometimes referred to as healing by primary intention. Chronic wounds are also sometimes referred to as healing by secondary intention. Granulation tissue at the base of the wound is generally of a greater size and healing also involves contraction of the wound through myofibroblasts (specialised cells in the granulation tissue) (Gould, 2001). Chronic wounds may have necrotic tissue and slough present. Necrotic tissue is dead tissue and is dark brown or black in colour. As it dries it forms a thick, black crust that is referred to as eschar. Slough is yellow fibrous tissue that is found on the surface of the wound bed. It is thought to be associated with bacterial activity (Thomas, 2000).

Microbiology and infection of wounds
Bacteria associated with acute wounds tend to be those that are common causes of wound infection including:

- *Staphylococcus aureus* (including MRSA)
- Enterobacteriaceae
- Coagulase-negative staphylococci
- *Pseudomonas* spp.
- Enterococci (Health Protection Agency, 2006)

Chronic wounds are generally colonised (up to 98%) with bacteria including:

- Coagulase-negative staphylococci
- *Staphylococcus aureus*
- ß-haemolytic streptococci
- *Streptococcus viridans*
- *Corynebacterium* spp.
- *Escherichia coli*
- *Klebsiella pneumoniae*
- *Enterobacter aerogenes*
- *Proprionibacterium acnes* (Bowler *et al.*, 1999)

Bacteria in chronic wounds may be associated with delayed wound healing as they can interfere with the formation of granulation tissue and may decrease collagen formation (Benbow, 2003). Colonising bacteria can become pathogenic in chronic wounds.

IDENTIFYING WOUND INFECTION

Wound infection is determined by the presence of clinical symptoms of infection with or without the presence of identified micro-organisms. The presence of micro-organisms alone in a wound is not an indicator of wound infection. Signs and symptoms of infection in acute wounds include:

- Redness
- Oedema
- Pain
- Wound exudate
- Heat around the wound
- Pus
- Abscess formation
- Pyrexia
- Raised white cell count in the absence of other foci of infection (Branom, 2002)

Signs and symptoms of infection in chronic wounds can be more subtle and less obvious. Wound infection should be considered if there is evidence of:

- Increase in exudate
- Increase in odour
- Increase in pain
- Slowing of healing
- Friable granulation tissue
- Wound breakdown
- Pocketing at the wound base
- Bridging of the epithelium (Cutting, 1998; Benbow, 2003)

Sampling wounds for micro-organisms can be undertaken in a number of ways. The commonest method is swabbing. The procedure for obtaining wound swabs is detailed in Chapter 3.

Other methods of wound sampling include punch biopsy, irrigation–aspiration and curettage. Whilst biopsies and curettage may be more accurate in identifying bacteria that are likely to be causing infection in chronic wounds, they are not as easy to perform as wound swabbing or irrigation–aspiration. Wound swabbing is a useful technique for identifying bacteria causing infection in acute wounds and if chronic wounds are cleansed of surface bacteria, swabs can still be a useful method of sampling bacteria in chronic wounds (McGuckin *et al.*, 2003). Whichever method of sampling is used, specimens should not be sent if there is no evidence of infection.

Preventing wound infection
The prevention of infection in acute surgical wounds in covered in Chapter 12. For acute traumatic wounds, prevention of infection involves cleansing of the wound to remove debris. Antibiotic therapy may be considered for some traumatic wounds, for example dog bites. Prevention of infection in chronic wounds involves good wound management and ensuring patient factors that increase risk of general infection are addressed, for example poor nutritional state.

TECHNIQUES FOR WOUND DRESSING
An aseptic technique is one that prevents micro-organisms from being transmitted, either directly or indirectly, to wounds (Bree-Williams and Waterman, 1996). Only sterile objects or fluids should come into contact with the wound during an aseptic technique. A clean technique is modified from an aseptic technique in that sterile equipment may not be used, but a non-touch technique is used (Infection Control Nurses Association, 2003). Traditionally, it has been assumed that an aseptic technique is used for acute wound healing by primary intention and that a clean technique can be used for chronic wound healing by secondary intention. However, it is important that a risk assessment is undertaken by an appropriately trained healthcare worker as to what technique is appropriate for wound management on an individual patient (Infection Control Nurses Association, 2003). The risk assessment must take into account the patient's risk of infection, for example an immunocompromised patient with a

chronic wound would require an aseptic technique. The location in which the patient is cared for must also be considered, for example if the patient with a chronic wound is on a ward where levels of MRSA are high then it might also be appropriate to use an aseptic technique.

Aseptic technique

The following general principles should be applied to aseptic techniques for wound dressings:

- Appropriate sterile equipment is available. The outer packaging of equipment should be intact and dry. The date of expiry should be checked.

- The setting is prepared. Aseptic techniques should not take place when dust creating activities (e.g. bedmaking and cleaning) are being carried out in the immediate vicinity. All equipment, for example dressing trolleys, should be checked for cleanliness and cleaned if necessary.

- The correct number of personnel are available to assist in the procedure.

- The relevant protective clothing is used:

  — For an aseptic technique sterile gloves should be worn. Whilst some local protocols may recommend the use of non-sterile gloves the evidence that it is safe to use non-sterile gloves for dressing acute wounds is lacking (St Clair and Larrabee, 2002) and there is evidence that examination gloves may be contaminated with micro-organisms before use (Berthelot *et al.*, 2006).

  — Aprons should be worn if there is risk of body fluid splash to clothing during the procedure, for example if wound irrigation is planned. The wearing of a plastic apron may also reduce risk of transfer of micro-organisms from uniform clothing during the procedure. If plastic aprons are worn for aseptic technique they should be stored in a clean location and not in the sluice, as storage in a designated dirty area can lead to contamination of clean aprons (Callaghan, 1998).

- Hand decontamination is observed. Alcohol hand gel is useful for rapid hand decontamination before, during and after an aseptic technique; free-standing bottles of alcohol hand gel can be taken to the patient's bedside on the bottom of the dressing trolley (Infection Control Nurses Association, 2003).

The following procedure can be followed if carrying out an aseptic technique, with or without the use of forceps:

(1) Prepare equipment. Clean trolley if necessary. Place dressing equipment and alcohol hand gel on bottom shelf of trolley and decontaminate hands.
(2) Prepare the dressing area. Close windows; ensure no cleaning or bedmaking activities are taking place. Pull curtains around bed. If using a treatment room, ensure that all surfaces are clean and dry.
(3) Prepare the patient. Explain the procedure and place the patient in a position that is comfortable for them and for the person who will be doing the dressing procedure.
(4) Take dressing trolley to bedside.
(5) Cleanse hands and loosen the existing dressing.
(6) Cleanse hands and open dressing pack on top surface of the trolley, taking care not to contaminate the inside of the pack.
(7) Carefully insert hand inside the yellow sterile bag and arrange the contents of the dressing pack as required on the sterile field.
(8) With hand still inside the yellow bag, use this to grasp and remove the existing dressing. Turn the bag over the dressing and attach to the side of the dressing trolley, with the removed dressing now inside.
(9) Add any additional items, for example cleansing solutions or new dressing.
(10) Decontaminate hands.
(11) Apply sterile gloves if using a gloved technique.
(12) Cleanse the wound using the appropriate technique, either irrigation or saline moistened gauze swabs.
(13) If using forceps, ensure that where these are used in contact with the wound or skin they do not contaminate sterile items when returning them to the trolley.

(14) Apply dressing.
(15) Dispose of waste into clinical waste bag and seal using the adhesive strip.
(16) Ensure the patient is made comfortable.
(17) Return the trolley to the preparation area, disposing of the small clinical waste bag into a larger bag before returning to the room.
(18) Clean trolley if necessary and decontaminate hands.
(19) Document procedure in patient records.

Clean technique
A clean technique can be performed using the above procedure, but using non-sterile gloves instead of sterile gloves. For a clean technique, a dressing trolley may not be needed; a procedure tray may be used as the surface on which to place the dressing field.

Wound cleansing solutions
The use of antiseptic solutions is no longer recommended for acute and chronic wound cleansing as some products have been shown to delay wound healing (Brennan and Leaper, 1985). However, where dressing techniques are being carried out at exit sites of invasive devices an antiseptic may be needed for cleansing, as a reduction in the number of micro-organisms at the site will be useful in preventing infection by migration of micro-organisms along the invasive device surface. Cleansing of the wound is only recommended if there is a need to remove excess exudate, dressing material, slough of necrosis. In particular, acute wounds should not be cleansed unless absolutely essential as the wound exudate contains healing factors (Vowden and Vowden, 2003). Cleansing solutions should be warmed to body temperature before use as reducing the wound temperature can delay wound healing (Johnson, 1987). Tap water has been recommended for cleansing traumatic wounds (Whaley, 2004) and for chronic wounds in the community (Selim *et al.*, 2001). The evidence that tap water is safe for cleansing of acute wounds is lacking (Patel and Beldon, 2003). The patient's intrinsic risk factors for infection and the quality of the water supply must be taken into consideration when determining whether tap water is safe to use for wound cleansing.

MANAGING INFECTED WOUNDS

If wound assessment indicates infection then an assessment should be made as to whether the patient requires systemic antibiotics. The choice of antibiotic will be dependent on:

- The microbial activity of the antibiotics available
- Patient allergies to antibiotics
- Penetration of the antibiotic into the tissues; this is important for deep-seated infections, such as osteomyelitis
- Other patient factors, for example do they have poor renal function that might affect their ability to metabolise and excrete the drug? (McGuckin *et al.*, 2003)

In addition to systemic therapy, management of the infected wound should focus on:

- Improving the patient's immune function
- Increasing vascular flow to the wound
- Removing dead tissue
- Controlling pain
- Managing exudate and odour by the appropriate dressing choice
- Healing the wound (Benbow, 2003)

The use of topical antimicrobial therapy for infected wounds is controversial. Antimicrobial dressings impregnated with silver and povidone iodine are available and may help to reduce levels of bacteria at the wound surface (Benbow, 2003). Evidence to support the widespread use of antimicrobial dressings for the treatment of infected wounds is currently lacking (Bergin and Wraight, 2006).

SUMMARY

The presence of a wound places patients at risk of infection due to the breach in the body's skin defence. Wound infection can delay the healing process as well as lead to more serious bloodstream infections. Preventing infection in wound management consists of good wound dressing technique and addressing factors that improve wound healing and immune function.

SCENARIO

Mrs Griffin is a 45-year-old lady who had an abdominal hysterectomy four days ago. She has a pyrexia of 38.6°C and the area around the wound appears inflamed. What are the requirements for her care at this stage?

A clinical assessment of the evidence of wound infection should be carried out and documented. If there is evidence of infection then antibiotics should be considered. As it is an acute surgical wound, one of the most likely causes is *Staphylococcus aureus*; therefore, any antibiotic prescribed should be effective against these bacteria. A wound swab can be taken and sent to the microbiology laboratory. The request form should indicate that this is a surgical wound and infection is suspected. If antibiotics are commenced before the swab is taken, these should also be noted on the request form. Wound dressings should be performed using an aseptic technique.

Wound infection is not determined by the presence of micro-organisms in wounds but by a clinical assessment for signs and symptoms of infection. Treatment of infected wounds will often be with systemic antimicrobials but should also include more holistic aspects, such as improving blood flow to the wound.

REFERENCES

Benbow, M. (2003) Managing infected wounds. *Nurse2Nurse Magazine*, **3** (6), 48–49.

Bergin, S.M. and Wraight, P. (2006) Silver based wound dressings and topical agents for treating diabetic foot ulcers. *Cochrane Database of Systematic Reviews 2006*. Available at: http://www.mrw.interscience.wiley.com/cochrane/clsysrev/articles/CD005082/pdf_fs.html (accessed 26 November 2006).

Berthelot, P., Dietemann, J., Fascia, P. *et al.* (2006) Bacterial contamination of non-sterile disposable gloves before use. *American Journal of Infection Control*, **34**, 128–130.

Bowler, P.G. and Davies, B.J. (1999) The microbiology of acute and chronic wounds. *Wounds*, **11** (4), 72–78.

Branom, R.N. (2002) Is this wound infected? *Critical Care Nursing Quarterly*, **25** (1), 55–62.

Bree-Williams, F.J. and Waterman, H. (1996) An examination of nurses' practices when performing aseptic technique for wound dressings. *Journal of Advanced Nursing*, **23**, 48–54.

Brennan, S.S. and Leaper, D.J. (1985) The effect of antiseptics on the healing wound: a study using the rabbit ear chamber. *British Journal of Surgery*, **72** (10), 780–782.

Callaghan, I. (1998) Bacterial contamination of nurses' uniforms: a study. *Nursing Standard*, **13** (1), 37–42.

Cutting, K. (1998) The causes and prevention of maceration of the skin. *Journal of Wound Care*, **8**, 200–201.

Gould, D. (2001) Clean surgical wounds: prevention of infection. *Nursing Standard*, **15** (49), 45–56.

Health Protection Agency (2006) *Surveillance of Surgical Site Infection in England: October 1997–September 2005.* Health Protection Agency, London.

Infection Control Nurses Association (2003) *Asepsis: Preventing Healthcare Associated Infection.* Infection Control Nurses Association, Bathgate.

Johnson, A. (1987) Wound healing under the microscope. *Nursing Times*, **83** (2), 12–15.

McGuckin, M., Goldman, R., Bolton, L. and Salcido, R. (2003) The clinical relevance of microbiology in acute and chronic wounds. *Advances in Skin and Wound Care*, **16** (1), 12–23.

Patel, S. and Beldon, P. (2003) Examining the literature on using tap water in wound cleansing. *Nursing Times*, **99** (43), 22–24.

Selim, P., Bashford, C. and Grossman, C. (2001) Evidence based practice: tap water cleansing in the community. *Journal of Clinical Nursing*, **10**, 372–379.

St Clair, K. and Larrabee, J.H. (2002) Clean versus sterile gloves: which to use for post-operative dressing changes? *Outcomes Management*, **6** (1), 17–21.

Thomas, S. (2000) Sterile maggots and the preparation of the wound bed. In: *Wound Bed Preparation. Proceedings of a Symposium Sponsored by the European Tissue Repair Society* (eds G.W. Cherry, K.G. Harding and T.J. Ryan). Royal Society of Medicine Press Ltd, Oxford.

Vowden, K. and Vowden, P. (2003) Understanding exudate management and the role of exudate in the healing process. *British Journal of Community Nursing*, **8** (11), 4–13.

Whaley, S. (2004) Tap water of normal saline for cleansing traumatic wounds. *British Journal of Community Nursing*, **9** (11), 471–478.

Control of Infection in Paediatric Settings

11

INTRODUCTION

The principles of infection prevention and control still apply to the care of children and babies; however, there are additional considerations, such as resident parents and siblings. Some infections are more common in these settings, for example specific respiratory viruses. This chapter covers the application of infection control principles within child and family centred care as well as infection prevention for specific paediatric infections.

LEARNING OBJECTIVES

By the end of this chapter you will be able to:

❑ Describe the application of infection prevention principles for children and babies
❑ Describe patient care and infection prevention requirements for infections common in children and babies

Babies and children can be affected by the same infections as adults in hospitals (e.g. MRSA and multi-resistant Gram negative bacteria) and the same basic principles for standard and isolation precautions apply. However, it is important in paediatric settings to apply these with reference to child and family centred care. Family centred care is 'a way of caring for children and their families within health services which ensures that care is planned around the whole family and not just the individual child/person, and in which all the family members are recognised as participants' (Shields *et al.*, 2006). The key principles of family centred care are:

- Incorporating the patient and family's knowledge, values, beliefs and cultural backgrounds into the planning and delivery of care
- Communicating timely, unbiased, complete and accurate information to patients and their families
- Encouraging and supporting patients and families to participate in care and decision making
- Involving patients and families in policy and programme design, healthcare facility design, professional education and delivery of care (Institute for Family Centred Care, 2006)

In applying these to infection control practice, there is a need to consider the additional role that parents and other carers will play in the nursing care of babies and children. They are likely to have more direct contact than with an adult through carrying out care activities and so will be more likely to be wearing protective clothing. This increased hands on care can also involve the care and management of invasive devices, such that their information and training needs will be greater and different. For small babies uniform and clothing can be contaminated in areas not generally considered to be important, for example the shoulders; appropriate protective clothing in the paediatric settings must address this. The wearing of protective clothing such as masks may scare children, but this must not compromise the precautions that staff take to protect themselves.

The personal and knowledge development of children is important and wherever possible the paediatric hospital setting must facilitate this. From an infection control perspective this means carefully considering whether isolation in a single room is essential, as social skills are an important part of childhood development. Therefore, restricting social contact can be detrimental. Play is also a vital part of childhood development. From this perspective children from different ward areas can mix in communal areas, leading to the risk of more widespread outbreaks of infection, such as diarrhoea and vomiting. Toys can also harbour micro-organisms and as such their decontamination needs to be addressed alongside decontamination of healthcare equipment.

Children are naturally inquisitive; therefore, the environment must be designed for their safety. Whereas in an adult setting it may be advisable to have sharps bins located close to the point of delivery of care, sharps bins must be located out of the reach of children. Cleaning and disinfection products, such as alcohol hand gel may also need careful consideration as to their location to ensure they are out of reach of children and not located at eye level. In paediatric settings, it may be prudent for individual staff to carry small bottles of gel rather than have wall mounted bottles. For all these reasons, infection prevention and control in paediatric settings demands additional considerations in terms of planning and management.

USE AND MANAGEMENT OF THE PLAYROOM

- Children should not attend communal play sessions if they are suffering from infectious conditions.
- Children colonised with antibiotic resistant organisms should not attend the playroom at the same time as children who are immunocompromised.
- The playroom should have appropriate hand hygiene facilities.
- The playroom should be on a schedule for regular cleaning.
- Records of children and siblings using the playroom per session could be useful in the event of contact tracing for an infectious disease.

INFECTION CONTROL RELATED TO TOYS

Toys can be a source of micro-organisms (Avila-Aguero *et al.*, 2003; Randle and Fleming, 2006) and in a hospital environment should be considered as communal patient equipment in the same manner as other healthcare related equipment. Computerised and electronic game consoles could be a source of micro-organisms, as computer keyboards in hospitals have been found to be commonly contaminated with pathogenic micro-organisms (Neely and Sittig, 2002). The following principles should be applied to toys in hospital settings:

- Communal soft toys should not be in use; babies and children should only have their own dedicated soft toys.

- Babies and children with long-term hospital stays should have their own soft toys laundered regularly.
- Babies and children being isolated for infectious conditions should have their soft toys laundered and all other toys cleaned at the end of a period of isolation as part of a discharge clean.
- Wipeable soft toys should be used in communal play areas and these should be cleaned on a regular schedule.
- Bath toys should be stored dry. Bath toys should be sealed to ensure no water can enter or remain inside.
- Computers and electronic game consoles should be cleaned regularly.
- Computer keyboards can be covered with a wipeable cover to prevent contamination.
- Toys taken into the cubicles of babies and children being isolated for an infectious condition must be adequately decontaminated before use by other children.
- Outdoor sandpits should be kept covered and the sand cleaned regularly by sieving and rinsing with a weak chemical disinfectant.
- Water play equipment should be emptied and dried at the end of each day.
- Children's hands should be washed before and after handling sand, water and soft modelling materials, including doughs.
- Soft modelling materials, including doughs should be replaced regularly. (Community Practitioners and Health Visitors Association and Infection Control Nurses Association, 2002; Avila-Aguero *et al.*, 2003; Randle and Fleming, 2006)

THE MILK KITCHEN

Contamination of formula milk during preparation by parents can lead to the milk being an infection risk (Mimouni *et al.*, 2002; Scientific Panel on Biological Hazards, 2004). Outbreaks of infection have also been linked to the handling of feeds for preterm infants (Berthelot *et al.*, 2001). Breast milk can also be contaminated (Olver *et al.*, 2000; Behari *et al.*, 2004) and should be handled with the same precautions as blood (UK Health Departments, 1998). There is a need to ensure it is handled and stored correctly in neonatal and paediatric settings. Therefore, whether infants are being fed with breast milk or formula milk, which is being prepared and handled by either staff or parents, it is important that good food hygiene principles are applied. When referring to infant feeding equipment the term sterilising is often used for decontamination in cold solutions (e.g. Milton) and for small steam sterilisers. In general, only disinfection is achieved but for consistency the term 'sterilising' will continue to be used.

Formula feeds

The following principles should be applied to the preparation of formula feeds in hospital settings:

- Ready prepared feed should be used in preference to making up formula feeds.
- Sterile bottles should be used.
- Feed should, wherever possible, be reconstituted in designated facilities with air treatment to avoid environmental contamination.
- Hands should be washed before handling bottles and other feeding items.
- When mixing formula milk, boiled water at a temperature greater than 70°C should be dispensed to the required volume and then the correct amount of powder added, as recommended by the manufacturer.
- Prepared feeds should be rapidly cooled.
- Use the reconstituted feed immediately and discard any remaining formula milk after feeding.
- Formula milk should not be prepared in advance and stored if appropriate facilities (i.e. a milk kitchen with air handling and adequately trained staff) are not in place. (Community Practitioners and Health Visitors Association and Infection Control Nurses Association, 2003; Scientific Panel on Biological Hazards, 2004)

Breast milk

It is important for paediatric settings to have guidelines for collection, storage and administration of breast milk to prevent bacterial contamination of the milk and to reduce risk of blood borne viruses, by protecting staff and by ensuring that breast milk is fed to the correct baby. The following principles should be applied to handling of breast milk:

- Breast milk is considered to be a high risk fluid for transmission of blood borne viruses and should be handled using the same precautions as for handling blood.
- Blood borne viruses can pass from mother to baby in breast milk; reference should be made to hospital policy and guidelines if mothers with blood borne viruses, for example HIV, wish to breastfeed.
- Breast milk should be handled aseptically during collection, storage and administration. Hand hygiene before and after any handling is important.
- Equipment used for breast milk collection must be designated to individual mothers and sterilised between use if not disposable.
- Breast milk collection and storage items must cleaned or disinfected after each use.
- Bottles used for storing breast milk must be easily cleanable and resistant to cracking or chipping.
- Reusable breast milk collection bottles must be discarded if chipped or scratched.
- Reusable breast milk storage bottles should be sterile at the point of use.
- Containers for breast milk should be clearly labelled with sufficient details to identify the mother and/or baby, the date and time of collection and should clearly state that the content is breast milk.
- Expressed breast milk should be used within two hours if kept at room temperature.
- Expressed breast milk can be kept refrigerated for up to 48 hours.
- Expressed breast milk can be kept frozen for up six months for well babies and up to three months for sick preterm babies.
- Designated refrigerators and freezers must be used for breast milk storage; it must not be stored with specimens, drugs or food.

- If a refrigerator is to be used for storage of both breast and formula milk, the breast milk should be placed in a plastic tray and stored at the bottom of the fridge.
- Refrigerators must be maintained at between 1–4°C. The temperature should be monitored daily and a record kept. Alarmed refrigerators are preferable.
- Freezers must be maintained at −18°C. The temperature should be monitored daily and a record kept. Alarmed freezers are preferable.
- Frozen breast milk should, out of preference, be thawed at room temperature or in a refrigerator. If it is necessary to thaw frozen milk rapidly using cool or warm water, care must be taken that water does not enter the bottle through the cap.
- Prior to feeding, a check should be made that the correct breast milk is being fed to the baby.
- If breast milk is fed to the wrong baby this must be treated as a contamination incident and the hospital policy followed in terms of blood borne virus testing and follow up. (UK Health Departments, 1998; UK Association of Milk Banks, 2001)

PREVENTION AND CONTROL OF SPECIFIC INFECTIONS

RESPIRATORY SYNCYTIAL VIRUS BRONCHIOLITIS

Respiratory syncytial virus (RSV) belongs to the Paramyxoviridae family and is a common cause of respiratory tract infection in both adults and children. It affects 90% of children in the first two years of life and is seasonal in that in temperate climates, such as that in the UK, most cases are seen during the winter season between November and February (Thorburn *et al.*, 2004).

Clinical symptoms of lower respiratory tract infection are more likely to be seen in babies under three months, premature births and babies with chronic conditions including congenital heart disease, cystic fibrosis, bronchopulmonary dysplasia, babies with a family history of asthma or atopic conditions such as eczema and babies living in low socio-economic conditions with exposure to passive smoking (Hawker *et al.*, 2005). Signs and symptoms of disease include:

- Rhinitis
- Cough
- Low grade pyrexia
- Croup
- Bronchiolitis with wheeze
- Otitis media (in approximately one third of children)
- Difficulty feeding
- Dyspnoea
- Pneumonia
- Apnoea (particularly in babies less than two months of age or who are preterm)

Transmission is by direct inhalation of airborne infectious droplets or from inoculation of the eyes or mucous membranes from contaminated surfaces. The virus can survive on inanimate objects, such as table tops and door handles for up to 24 hours and on gowns, hands and tissues for up to one hour (Hawker *et al.*, 2005). The incubation period is from 2–8 days but is most commonly 4–6 days. Babies and children are infectious from up to three days before onset of symptoms until respiratory symptoms cease; however, the virus may still be shed in young babies for up to four weeks.

In addition to standard precautions, the following infection control precautions should be applied (Karanfil *et al.*, 1999; Thorburn *et al.*, 2004; Hawker *et al.*, 2005).

Patient placement
Symptomatic children should be isolated in a single room with the door closed, regardless of whether RSV has been confirmed, as other respiratory viruses, for example para-influenza, could be causing the symptoms.

Where wards have more than one child with the infection they may be cohorted together in an area in which the door can be closed.

Staff
There is no restriction on staff that can care for RSV positive children.

Where possible, staff caring for an RSV positive child should not look after any other children. Where this is not possible they must not be allocated to look after other babies and children who are immunocompromised or who have heart or lung defects.

Specimens
Nasopharyngeal secretions should be sent to the laboratory for diagnosis.

Treatment
Treatment is dependent on the severity of disease and may include:

- Oxygen
- Upper airway suctioning
- Mechanical ventilation
- Nebulised salbutamol
- Ribavarin

Prophylaxis
Palivizumab prophylaxis should be considered for:

- Children under two years of age with chronic lung disease, on home oxygen or who have had prolonged oxygen use
- Infants less than six months of age who have left to right shunt haemodynamically significant congenital heart disease and/or pulmonary hypertension
- Children under two years of age with severe congenital immunodeficiency (Joint Committee on Vaccination and Immunisation, 2005)

Protective clothing
All staff having direct contact with the child or their immediate surroundings should wear disposable aprons or gowns.

Hand hygiene
Hands should be decontaminated with either hand washing or use of alcohol hand gel before and after any contact with the child

as well as on removal of protective clothing. Hands should be decontaminated on leaving the cubicle or cohort area.

Cleaning procedures
Good daily cleaning with a disinfectant, for example hypochlorite, is important to remove environmental viral contamination.

Discharge cleaning
A thorough clean with a disinfectant, for example hypochlorite, is required. Curtains should be changed and laundered.

Equipment
Wherever possible equipment should be dedicated to the isolation room or cohort area. Reusable equipment must be adequately decontaminated before using on another patient (refer to Chapter 16).

Crockery and cutlery may be washed in the dishwasher in the usual manner.

Waste
Treat as clinical waste.

Linen
Treat linen as infected.

Transfers to other wards and departments
Patients with RSV should not be transferred to other wards unless it is clinically necessary or for the purpose of isolation or cohorting. They should not use the playroom whilst they are symptomatic.

Visits to other departments, such as radiology, should be kept to a minimum. Where visits are necessary the receiving department must be told in advance and the following principles applied:

- Transporting staff, for example porters, should wear disposable aprons and gloves only when they are in contact with the child; these should be discarded immediately contact has ceased.

- Hand hygiene by hand washing or alcohol gel is necessary after child and equipment contact.
- Trolleys or pushchairs used for transfers should be decontaminated before use on another child.
- Children should not wait in holding areas with other children, wherever possible, but should be brought to the department immediately before and returned to their isolation room immediately after treatments or investigations.

Visitors
Relatives with signs of active respiratory infection should be discouraged from visiting. Protective clothing should be worn by parents and carers when they are assisting in care during which they are likely to be contaminated with nasopharyngeal secretions, for example wiping noses. The family should be encouraged to remain in the child's room wherever possible and instructed not to have contact with other parents and children on the ward. All visitors should be instructed on the precautions required, including hand hygiene on leaving the room.

Discharge
No specific precautions are needed.

Deceased children
No specific precautions are required.

VARICELLA ZOSTER VIRUS (CHICKENPOX)
Chickenpox is the primary infection with varicella zoster virus. It is an acute illness that is characterised by the classical skin rash of vesicular lesions. The route of spread is by the airborne route or from contact with vesicle fluid; contact with vesicle fluid from a shingles rash (the latent form of the virus) can cause chickenpox in someone who is non-immune. Chickenpox starts with a generalised viral syndrome (malaise and fever) before the appearance of the skin lesions. The lesions typically appear in successive crops, over a period of up to several days. The number of lesions can range from a few, to extensive coverage of the body. In some cases, the disease is so mild, with few lesions, that it is not noticed.

The incubation period ranges from 8–21 days, but illness is typically noted between 13 and 17 days. The infectious period is from three days before the spots develop until seven days after the appearance of the last crop of spots, but the period of infectivity can be prolonged in immunocompromised children. The disease can be very severe in children who are immunocompromised. In neonates who develop the disease within ten days of birth, or whose mothers develop chickenpox between five days before and two days after birth, the risk of severe disease is high, with an increased mortality rate. Immunity after infection is generally lifelong, but will be reduced for those whose immune systems are compromised by disease or medication. Immunity passes from mother to child; therefore babies whose mothers are immune to chickenpox are also likely to be immune up to six months of age. Babies who are born before 28 weeks of gestation or whose birth weight is less that 1000 g may not acquire maternal antibodies (UK Health Departments, 2006); babies who have received exchange blood transfusions, for example during cardiac bypass surgery, may also lose maternal antibody immunity.

Due to the infectivity and severe consequences in those with altered immunity and neonates, contact tracing and assessment of immune status is necessary when a case of chickenpox is identified in in-patient children or in staff. When this occurs the infection control team for the hospital should be notified immediately as there is limited time in which to carry out contact tracing and immunity testing. For babies and neonates most at risk of severe disease, passive immunity in the form of varicella zoster immunoglobulin will be considered. This has to be given within eight days of exposure to chickenpox, hence the need for prompt action.

The following infection control measures should be applied to the care of a child with chickenpox in hospital (Hawker *et al.*, 2005).

Patient placement
Children with chickenpox must be isolated in a single room with the door closed until seven days after the eruption of the last crop of spots.

On wards with immunocompromised children, for example renal and oncology wards, a negative pressure isolation room should be used. A negative pressure room is specifically designed and maintained so that the air pressure outside the room is higher than the air pressure in the room. When the door is opened the difference in pressure means that air from outside the room is drawn in so that there is no risk of droplets of varicella zoster releasing from the room. Air is extracted from the room either through a filter or is discharged from a location where there is no risk of other patients coming into contact with the air extract. If a negative pressure room is not located on these wards then consideration should be given to moving the child to a ward where children are less likely to be at risk of severe infection.

Staff
Only staff known to be immune to chickenpox should have contact with children with chickenpox. Staff who have lowered immunity due to being on immunosuppressant therapy or on very high dose steroids should avoid contact.

Treatment
Supportive treatment is generally the only treatment given. Acyclovir may be considered in certain circumstances to lessen the symptoms of the disease.

Protective clothing
Gloves and aprons should be worn by all personnel having direct contact with the child or their immediate environment.

Hand hygiene
Hands should be decontaminated on entering and leaving the cubicle with either hand washing or with alcohol hand gel.

Cleaning procedures
This should be as for standard procedures for general cleaning. On discharge the room should be thoroughly cleaned with a disinfectant solution, for example hypochlorite, and the curtains changed.

Equipment

Wherever possible, equipment should be dedicated to the isolation room or cohort area. Reusable equipment must be adequately decontaminated before using on another patient (refer to Chapter 16).

Crockery and cutlery may be washed in the dishwasher in the usual manner.

Waste

Treat as clinical waste.

Linen

Treat linen as infected.

Transfers to other wards and departments

Patients with chickenpox should not be transferred to other wards unless it is clinically necessary or for the purpose of isolation. They should not use the playroom during their period of isolation.

Visits to other departments, such as radiology, should be kept to a minimum. Where visits are necessary, the receiving department must be told in advance and the following principles applied:

- Transporting staff and other staff in the receiving department should only have contact if they are immune to chickenpox.
- Transporting staff, for example porters, should wear disposable aprons and gloves only when they are in contact with the child; these should be discarded immediately contact has ceased.
- Hand hygiene by hand washing or alcohol gel is necessary after child and equipment contact.
- Trolleys or pushchairs used for transfers should be decontaminated before use on another child.
- Children must not wait in holding areas with other children, but must be brought to the department immediately before and returned to their isolation room immediately after treatments or investigations.

Visitors

Only relatives who have themselves had chickenpox should visit. Siblings who are not immune may also develop the disease, either from the same contact as the patient or from having had contact with the patient. Wherever possible they should be excluded from visiting and must not use communal areas of the hospital or ward, such as the playroom.

Protective clothing need not be worn by parents and carers if they are immune to chickenpox. The family should be encouraged to remain in the child's room wherever possible and instructed not to have contact with other parents and children on the ward. All visitors should be instructed on the precautions required, including hand hygiene on leaving the room.

Discharge

No specific precautions are needed.

Deceased children

No specific precautions are required.

MUMPS

Mumps is caused by a paramyxovirus and is also known as infectious parotitis. The disease is characterised by unilateral or bilateral facial swellings. Inflammation of the testes and ovaries can also occur in adolescents. The incubation period is from 12–25 days, but symptoms generally occur 16–18 days after exposure. Transmission is by the airborne route from droplets and by direct contact with the saliva of an infected person. The period of infectivity is from seven days before the onset of facial swelling to nine days after. Children who have been vaccinated, either through a combined vaccine or a single vaccine, should only be considered immune if they have received the full course.

Due to the infectivity, contact tracing and assessment of immune status is necessary when a case of mumps is identified in in-patient children or in staff. When this occurs the infection control team for the hospital should be notified immediately as there is limited time in which to carry out contact tracing and immunity testing.

The following infection control measures should be applied to the care of a child with mumps in hospital (Chin, 2000; Hawker *et al.*, 2005).

Patient placement
Children with mumps must be isolated in a single room with the door closed until nine days after the appearance of facial swelling.

Staff
Only staff known to be immune to mumps should have contact with children with mumps.

Treatment
Supportive treatment is generally the only treatment given.

Protective clothing
Gloves and aprons should be worn by all personnel having direct contact with the child or their immediate environment.

Hand hygiene
Hands should be decontaminated on entering and leaving the cubicle with either hand washing or with alcohol hand gel.

Cleaning procedures
These should be as for standard procedures for general cleaning. On discharge, the room should be thoroughly cleaned with a disinfectant solution, for example hypochlorite, and the curtains changed.

Equipment
Wherever possible equipment should be dedicated to the isolation room or cohort area. Reusable equipment must be adequately decontaminated before using on another patient (refer to Chapter 16).

Crockery and cutlery may be washed in the dishwasher in the usual manner.

Waste
Treat as clinical waste.

Linen
Treat linen as infected.

Transfers to other wards and departments
Patients with mumps should not be transferred to other wards unless it is clinically necessary or for the purpose of isolation. They should not use the playroom during their period of isolation.

Visits to other departments, such as radiology, should be kept to a minimum. Where visits are necessary the receiving department must be told in advance and the following principles applied:

- Transporting staff and other staff in the receiving department should only have contact if they are immune to mumps.
- Transporting staff, for example porters, should wear disposable aprons and gloves only when they are in contact with the child; these should be discarded immediately contact has ceased.
- Hand hygiene by hand washing or alcohol gel is necessary after child and equipment contact.
- Trolleys or pushchairs used for transfers should be decontaminated before use on another child.
- Children must not wait in holding areas with other children, but must be brought to the department immediately before and returned to their isolation room immediately after treatments or investigations.

Visitors
Only relatives who have themselves had mumps or are immune through vaccination should visit. Siblings who are not immune may also develop the disease, either from the same contact as the patient or from having had contact with the patient. Wherever possible they should be excluded from visiting and must not use communal areas of the hospital or ward, such as the playroom.

Protective clothing need not be worn by parents and carers if they are immune to mumps. The family should be encouraged to remain in the child's room wherever possible and instructed not to have contact with other parents and children on the ward. All visitors should be instructed on the precautions required, including hand hygiene on leaving the room.

Discharge
No specific precautions needed.

Deceased children
No specific precautions are required.

MEASLES
Measles is caused by a paramyxovirus. It is characterised by the appearance of Koplik spots on the mucosa of the cheeks, followed by a florid maculopapular rash that extends across the whole body. Pyrexia and upper respiratory symptoms, including cough and rhinitis precede the development of the rash. It is transmitted by the airborne route and by contact with the nasopharyngeal secretions of an infected person. The incubation period ranges from 7–18 days but is commonly 8–12 days. The period of infectivity is from three days before the onset of symptoms to five days after the appearance of the rash. Children who have been vaccinated, either through a combined vaccine or a single vaccine, should only be considered immune if they have received the full course.

Due to the infectivity, contact tracing and assessment of immune status is necessary when a case of measles is identified in in-patient children or in staff. When this occurs the infection control team for the hospital should be notified immediately as there is limited time in which to carry out contact tracing and immunity testing.

The following infection control measures should be applied to the care of a child with measles in hospital (Hawker *et al.*, 2005).

Patient placement
Children with measles must be isolated in a single room with the door closed until five days after the appearance of the rash.

Staff
Only staff known to be immune to measles should have contact with children with measles.

Treatment
Supportive treatment is generally the only treatment given.

Protective clothing
Gloves and aprons should be worn by all personnel having direct contact with the child or their immediate environment.

Hand hygiene
Hands should be decontaminated on entering and leaving the cubicle, with either hand washing or with alcohol hand gel.

Cleaning procedures
These should be as for standard procedures for general cleaning. On discharge, the room should be thoroughly cleaned with a disinfectant solution, for example hypochlorite, and the curtains changed.

Equipment
Wherever possible, equipment should be dedicated to the isolation room or cohort area. Reusable equipment must be adequately decontaminated before using on another patient (refer to Chapter 16).

Crockery and cutlery may be washed in the dishwasher in the usual manner.

Waste
Treat as clinical waste.

Linen
Treat linen as infected.

Transfers to other wards and departments
Patients with measles should not be transferred to other wards unless it is clinically necessary or for the purpose of isolation. They should not use the playroom during their period of isolation.

Visits to other departments, such as radiology, should be kept to a minimum. Where visits are necessary the receiving department must be told in advance and the following principles applied:

- Transporting staff and other staff in the receiving department should only have contact if they are immune to measles.
- Transporting staff, for example porters, should wear disposable aprons and gloves only when they are in contact with the child; these should be discarded immediately contact has ceased.
- Hand hygiene by hand washing or alcohol gel is necessary after child and equipment contact.
- Trolleys or pushchairs used for transfers should be decontaminated before use on another child.
- Children must not wait in holding areas with other children, but must be brought to the department immediately before and returned to their isolation room immediately after treatments or investigations.

Visitors

Only relatives who have themselves had measles or are immune by vaccination should visit. Siblings who are not immune may also develop the disease, either from the same contact as the patient or from having had contact with the patient. Wherever possible they should be excluded from visiting and must not use communal areas of the hospital or ward, such as the playroom.

Protective clothing need not be worn by parents and carers if they are immune to measles. The family should be encouraged to remain in the child's room wherever possible and instructed not to have contact with other parents and children on the ward. All visitors should be instructed on the precautions required, including hand hygiene on leaving the room.

Discharge

No specific precautions are needed.

Deceased children

No specific precautions are required.

OTHER CHILDHOOD INFECTIOUS CONDITIONS

Brief information on transmission routes, incubation periods and infection control measures for other common childhood infections is given in Table 11.1.

Table 11.1 Common childhood infectious conditions and infection control measures (Hawker et al., 2005).

Disease/organism	Incubation period	Clinical features	Mode of transmission	Infection control measures
Adenovirus	4–5 days	Pyrexia, sore throat, rhinitis	Contact with respiratory secretions	Standard precautions. Isolation not required.
Rotavirus	1–3 days	Sudden onset diarrhoea and vomiting with mild pyrexia	Faecal-oral route and through contaminated water	Isolation required until 48 hours after cessation of symptoms.
Hand foot and mouth disease (Coxsackie virus)	3–5 days	Small lesions inside the mouth and throat and on the palms, fingers and soles of feet	Contact with respiratory secretions	Standard precautions. Isolation not required.
Ringworm	2–38 weeks	First appears as a small red spot, which, as it grows, the centre heals, leaving the classic ring-like appearance	Contact, either directly or with contaminated objects, including combs	Standard precautions. Isolation may be required in certain units where patients are immunocompromised.
Impetigo	Variable		Contact	Isolation may be required in high risk units.
Rubella		Rash preceded by fever and upper respiratory symptoms	Contact with respiratory secretions and droplet	Isolation required.
Slapped cheek (Parvovirus)	13–18 days	Maculopapular rash on limbs and trunk with bright red cheeks	Airborne by droplet	Isolation required in units where patients are immunocompromised. Contact with pregnant healthcare workers should be avoided.
Whooping cough (pertussis)	7–10 days	Cough, cold and pyrexia that becomes paroxysmal with bouts of coughing	Airborne by droplet	Isolation required.

SCENARIO

Jack is a five-year-old boy who is admitted with an acute exacerbation of asthma. The following day he develops a vesicular rash that is diagnosed as being chickenpox. What are the specific infection control precautions that should now be put in place?

Jack should be moved to a single room and the door should be kept closed. Only staff that are immune to chickenpox should provide his care. His parents should be asked to ensure that only visitors who are known to have had chickenpox visit. Jack should be excluded from the play and communal areas. The infection control team should be advised, as the immune status of staff and patients contacts will need to be checked.

SUMMARY

Paediatric settings can provide challenges in infection prevention and control due to the involvement of the family in aspects of care. Many of the infections relevant in this setting are viral in nature. Infection prevention practices apply not only to the care setting but also to play and recreational activities.

REFERENCES

Avila-Aguero, M.L., German, G., Paris, M.M., Hererra, J.F. and the Safe Toy Study Group (2003) Toys in a pediatric hospital: are they a bacterial source? *American Journal of Infection Control*, **32**, 287–290.

Behari, P., England, J., Alscaid, G., Garcia-Houchins, S. and Weber, S. (2004) Transmission of meticillin resistant staphylococcus aureus to preterm infants through breast milk. *Infection Control and Hospital Epidemiology*, **25** (9), 778–780

Berthelot, P., Grattard, F., Pataral, H. *et al.* (2001) Nosocomial colonisation of premature babies with *Klebsiella oxytoca*: probable role of enteral feeding procedure in transmission and control of the outbreak with the use of gloves. *Infection Control and Hospital Epidemiology*, **22**, 148–151.

Chin, J. (2000) *Control of Communicable Disease.* American Public Health Association, Washington, DC.

Community Practitioners and Health Visitors Association and Infection Control Nurses Association (2002) *Keep it Clean and Healthy: Infection Control Guidance for Playgroups and other Childcare Settings.* Pat Cole, Hartford.

Community Practitioners and Health Visitors Association and Infection Control Nurses Association (2003) *Looking after You and Your*

Baby: a CPHVA and ICNA Guide to Health and Hygiene for Parents and Others Caring for Babies. Pat Cole, Hartford.

Hawker, J., Begg, N., Blair, I., Reintjes, R. and Weinberg, J. (2005) *Communicable Disease Control Handbook.* Blackwell Publishing, Oxford.

Institute for Family Centred Care (2006) Patient and family centred care. Available at: http://www.familycenteredcare.org/ (accessed 23 November 2006).

Joint Committee on Vaccination and Immunisation (2005) *Meeting Minutes 22 June 2005.* Available at: http://www.advisorybodies.doh.gov.uk/jcvi/mins220605.htm (accessed 26 November 2006).

Karanfil, L.V., Conlon, M., Lykrens, K. *et al.* (1999) Reducing the rate of nosocomially transmitted respiratory syncytial virus. *American Journal of Infection Control*, **27** (2), 91–96.

Mimouni, F.B., Inbar, M. and Dollberg, S. (2002) Bacterial contamination during routine formula preparation. *American Journal of Infection Control*, **30**, 44–45.

Neely, A.N. and Sittig, D.F. (2002) Basic microbiologic and infection control information to reduce the potential transmission of pathogens to patients via computer hardware. *Journal of the American Medical Information Association*, **9**, 500–508.

Olver, W.J., Bond, D.W., Boswell, T.C. and Watkin, S.L. (2000) Neonatal group B streptococcal disease associated with infected breast milk. *Archives of Disease in Childhood*, **83**, F48–49.

Randle, J. and Fleming, K. (2006) The risk of infection from toys in the intensive care setting. *Nursing Standard*, **20**, 50–54.

Scientific Panel on Biological Hazards (2004) Opinion of the Scientific Panel on Biological Hazards on a request from the Commission related to microbiological risks in infant formulae and follow-on formulae. *European Food Safety Association Journal*, **113**, 1–35.

Shields, L., Pratt, J. and Hunter, J. (2006) Family centred care: a review of qualitative studies. *Journal of Clinical Nursing*, **15** (10), 1317–1323.

Thorburn, K., Kerr, S., Taylor, N. and van Saene, H.K.F. (2004) RSV outbreak in a paediatric intensive care unit. *Journal of Hospital Infection*, **57**, 194–201.

UK Association of Milk Banks (2001) *Guidelines for the Collection, Storage and Handling of Breast Milk for a Mother's Own Baby in Hospital* (second edition). UK Association of Milk Banks, London.

United Kingdom Health Departments (1998) *Guidance for Clinical Healthcare Workers: Protection Against Infection With Blood Borne Viruses.* The Stationery Office, London.

United Kingdom Health Departments (2006) *Immunisation Against Infectious Diseases.* The Stationery Office, London.

12 | Peri-operative Care Settings

INTRODUCTION
Patients in the peri-operative setting are particularly vulnerable to infection as their care and management often involves the use of multiple invasive devices as well as breaching their body defences through surgical incisions. A high standard of infection prevention is vital in this setting. This chapter covers infection prevention in the anaesthetic room, the operating room and the post-anaesthesia care unit.

LEARNING OBJECTIVES
By the end of this chapter you will be able to:

❏ Describe additional standard precaution requirements in this setting
❏ Discuss the particular infection prevention requirements for specific infections including:

— Meticillin resistant *Staphylococcus aureus*
— Tuberculosis
— Creutzfeldt-Jakob disease

INFECTION CONTROL IN ANAESTHESIA
Anaesthetic and post-anaesthetic care areas are part of the operating suite; therefore, the infection control practices need to reflect the increased need for asepsis in this area. Standard precautions should be applied in both of these areas. In addition to standard precautions, the following practices should be applied in anaesthetic and post-anaesthetic care:

• Theatre clothing should be worn in line with that required in the operating suite policy.

- Drugs should be prepared using an aseptic procedure.
- Single use ampoules should be discarded when the required amount of drug has been withdrawn.
- Multiple use vials must be stored correctly between use and the rubber bung decontaminated with an alcohol wipe before accessing.
- Maximal barrier precautions, including a full surgical hand wash and the wearing of a cap, mask, sterile gown and sterile gloves, together with the use of a large sterile drape should be applied to insertion of central lines and all spinal, epidural and caudal procedures.
- Sterile gloves must be worn following hand disinfection and a small sterile drape used for peripheral regional blocks and arterial line insertions.
- Insertion of peripheral cannulae requires an aseptic technique involving hand decontamination, skin preparation with an antiseptic solution and the wearing of non-sterile gloves. (Association of Anaesthetists of Great Britain and Ireland, 2002)

Management and care of epidural catheters

The insertion of epidural lines carries a risk of both superficial skin infection but also deep-seated infections that can have severe consequences for patients. Superficial infection rates range from 4.3–12% and deep infection rates have been found to be in the region of 0.3% (Holt *et al.*, 1995). The site at which the epidural is inserted affects the rate of infection, with thoracic sites being responsible for 44% of infections, lumbar 38% and cervical 6% (Ngan Kee *et al.*, 1992). The organisms most commonly responsible for epidural infection are:

- *Staphylococcus aureus*
- *Staphylococcus epidermidis*
- *Pseudomonas* spp.
- *Enterococci*

Micro-organisms can be introduced at the point of catheter or needle insertion. They can also migrate along the catheter from the exit site. Rarely, epidural associated infections can occur due to contaminated infusate. Superficial infection is characterised by erythema, oedema and pain around the insertion site, with or without the presence of purulent exudate. Deep infection is characterised by fever, neck stiffness, headache, vomiting, altered sensory or motor responses in the lower limbs and a decrease in efficacy of infused medication.

The following principles should be applied to insertion and management of epidural lines to reduce risk of infection:

- A sterile technique should be used for insertion that includes sterile gown, gloves, drapes and adequate skin preparation.
- An aseptic technique must be followed for all manipulations of the line.
- The line should not include any injection ports.
- A sterile dressing that allows inspection of the insertion site should be used. This should be inspected at least daily and changed using an aseptic technique if there is evidence of lifting, to expose the insertion site or leakage.
- The insertion site should be inspected daily for signs of superficial infection and the assessment documented.
- Infusates should be pre-prepared single use, or if being made up they should be prepared under strict aseptic conditions, preferably within a pharmacy department. (Dawson, 2001; Association of Anaesthetists of Great Britain and Ireland, 2002; Royal College of Nursing, 2005)

Decontamination of anaesthetic equipment

Anaesthetic equipment should be handled, decontaminated and stored in line with the principles described in Chapter 16. Decontamination of specific anaesthetic equipment is detailed in Table 12.1.

STANDARD INFECTION CONTROL PRECAUTIONS IN THE OPERATING THEATRE

In addition to universal and standard precautions in ward areas, the nature of operating department practice demands additional standard precautions. As well as the precautions described in Chapter 5, the following precautions apply to operating department settings:

Table 12.1 Decontamination of anaesthetic equipment.

Equipment	Decontamination process
Anaesthetic masks	Disposable single patient use or sterilisation.
Oral, nasopharyngeal and tracheal airways and tubes	Disposable single patient use.
Laryngeal masks	Single patient use preferable. Reusable masks should be at a minimum disinfected in a sterile services department. Most manufacturers stipulate a maximum number of decontamination processes. Records must be kept for each mask to ensure the maximum number of decontamination processes is not breached.
Breathing systems	Single patient use preferable. If used with a filter then they may be changed in accordance with manufacturers' instructions but preferably daily. Circuits used for more than one patient must be checked before each patient use for signs of visible contamination.
Anaesthetic machines	A bacterial/viral filter should be used to protect the machine from contamination. Surfaces of the machine should be cleaned on a daily basis and whenever visibly soiled. Tubing, bellows, carbon dioxide absorbers and unidirectional valves should be changed and decontaminated in accordance with manufacturers' instructions.
Laryngoscopes	Disposable single use blades are preferable. Reusable blades should be sterilised in a sterile services department. Handles should be decontaminated regularly by washing and disinfecting and always when visibly soiled.
Intubating bronchoscopes and flexible laryngoscopes	The fibre optic mechanism in these devices makes them unsuitable for sterilising by heat. They should undergo a cleaning and a high-level disinfection process before use wherever possible and always undergo these processes after each use. Disinfected scopes should be stored dry and protected from dust and contamination between uses.
Bougies	Manufacturers' recommendations for decontamination should be followed but a minimum of disinfection is required. Disinfected bougies should be stored dry and protected from dust and contamination between uses. Where manufacturers recommend a limited number of uses, a tracking system must be in place for each bougie to ensure the maximum use is not breached.
Oxygen masks and tubing	Disposable single patient use
Suction catheters	Disposable single patient use
Suction tubing	Disposable single patient use

- The patient should be prepared with a clean gown and bed/trolley linen before being transferred to the operating theatre.
- Only the minimum number of theatre staff should be in the operating theatre.
- There should be an effective air exchange system that delivers a minimum of 20 air changes per hour.
- Movement and talking should be restricted to the minimum in the operating theatre.
- The theatre doors should be kept closed to maintain the appropriate air pressures.
- Decontamination and disposal of equipment should be carried out in line with local policies.
- The operating table and all other patient contact surfaces should be decontaminated between cases.
- There should be effective communication between the operating theatre and ward areas to ensure the department is advised in advance of infectious cases.

Due to the nature of operating department work, there is greater risk of blood and body fluid contact, as well as of needlestick injuries. The following precautions should be applied to reduce this risk:

- Double gloving should be considered for all surgical procedures, but should be applied to all surgical procedures involving sharps and orthopaedic surgery.
- Change gloves regularly during prolonged procedures.
- If glove puncture is suspected or recognised, re-scrub and re-glove as soon as possible.
- Masks and goggles or a full face visor should be worn by members of the scrub team; the mask should be fluid repellent.
- Masks should be removed and discarded immediately after each operation or procedure and should not be left to hang around the neck of the wearer.
- Male healthcare workers should consider hoods to protect freshly shaven cheeks and necks.

- Wellingtons or calf-length boots should be considered if there is a risk of legs or feet becoming contaminated.
- Hand-to-mouth contact should be avoided.
- Eating and drinking should be prohibited, as should the application of cosmetics, lip balm and contact lenses in the clinical area.
- Appropriate devices should be used for applying and removing surgical blades.
- Avoid more than one person working in an open wound or body cavity at any one time.
- Use instruments rather than fingers for retraction and holding tissue.
- Sharps and sharp instruments should not be passed hand to hand; a neutral zone, for example a receiver, should be used for placement and retrieval.
- Do not leave instruments exposed in the operative field but remove to the neutral zone as soon as possible.
- A disposable device should be used for containing needles and sharps; this should be discarded into a sharps bin at the end of the procedure.
- Remove sharp suture needles before tying.
- Use blunt suture needles or staples where possible.
- Avoid using fingers to guide sharp suture needles.
- Opt for less invasive surgical procedures wherever possible.
- Collecting drapes should be used if there is a risk of excessive blood/body fluid loss, for example caesarean sections.
- Avoid the use of sharp clips for holding surgical drapes.
- The operating table should be protected with a non-permeable sheet.
- Fluid waste should be handled with care to prevent splashing.
- Closed system suction should be used.
- The patient's skin should be cleaned of all visible blood before leaving the operating theatre and bloodstained linen changed.
- Footwear should be decontaminated by the wearer after use. (UK Health Departments, 1998; Woodhead *et al.*, 2002; National Association of Theatre Nurses, 2004)

SURGICAL HAND PREPARATION PROCEDURE

The purpose of a surgical hand preparation procedure is to remove transient micro-organisms and to reduce levels of resident micro-organisms (National Association of Theatre Nurses, 2004). One of the following antiseptics is used for this purpose:

- Chlorhexidine gluconate
- Povidone iodine
- Triclosan

Prior to surgical hand preparation staff should ensure that hair is fully enclosed under a theatre hat/cap and that a new surgical face mask is correctly positioned over the nose and mouth and fits the wearer comfortably. Eye protection should be applied if appropriate. No wrist or hand jewellery should be worn, with the exception of a plain wedding band. Finger nails should be no longer than the fingertips as glove punctures may occur. Any cuts or abrasions on the hands or forearms should be covered with a waterproof dressing.

For surgical hand preparation the following procedure can be followed:

(1) Ensure all requirements, for example sterile nailbrush, gown pack, are ready for use.
(2) Turn on water and adjust temperature and spray.
(3) Wet the hands and forearms.
(4) Keeping the hands higher than the elbows throughout the wash and avoiding excess splashing, apply 2–3 ml of antiseptic agent from the dispenser using the elbow lever.
(5) Wash hands and forearms thoroughly up to 5 cm below the elbows for a minimum of one minute.
(6) Using a sterile nailbrush gently clean the nails for a minimum of 30 seconds per hand.
(7) Rinse thoroughly with running water.
(8) Keeping the hands higher than the elbows throughout the wash and avoiding excess splashing, apply a second 2–3 ml of antiseptic agent from the dispenser using the elbow lever.
(9) Wash hands and forearms to two thirds of the way down the forearm for a minimum of two minutes.

(10) Rinse thoroughly with running water.
(11) Keeping the hands higher than the elbows throughout the wash and avoiding excess splashing, apply a third 2–3 ml of antiseptic agent from the dispenser using the elbow lever.
(12) Wash hands to below wrists for a minimum of one minute.
(13) Rinse thoroughly with running water.
(14) Dry hands with sterile towels using a blotting technique from hand to elbow.

For subsequent scrubs it is acceptable to use a hand wash followed by the application of an alcoholic hand gel for hand preparation, provided the scrub team are moving directly from one procedure to another (National Association of Theatre Nurses, 2004). It is important that sufficient product is applied to cover all areas of the hands and forearms and a technique of application should be used to ensure all areas have contact with the alcoholic hand preparation.

GOWNING PROCEDURE

Sterile gowns are worn to prevent skin from the operator contaminating the operation site and to provide a barrier between sterile and unsterile areas. In addition, they are worn to protect the operator and scrub team from contact with the patient's blood and body fluids. The level of barrier protection provided by a surgical gown is determined by European Standard EN13795 (2002). Surgical gowns should comply with the following requirements:

• Resistance to bacterial penetration
• Resistance to liquid penetration
• Comfort for the wearer
• Practicality for theatre use
• Tensile strength (Multidisciplinary Working Group, 2003)

The following procedure can be followed when gowning in the operating theatre:

(1) Ensure the sterile gown pack is intact before use and this should be opened before the surgical scrub procedure commences.

(2) Paying attention so as not to drip excess water onto the sterile gown field, dry hands and arms carefully with the sterile hand towel using a rotating and blotting movement. One towel should be used for each arm.

(3) Lift the sterile gown off the sterile field and step back away from the trolley/field.

(4) Holding the inside of the gown below the neckline allow the gown to unfold, taking care that the gown does not touch the floor and only the inside of the gown is touched with bare hands.

(5) Don the gown by placing both arms into the sleeves together. Assistance in donning may be needed from the circulating practitioner.

(6) If using a closed method for gloving, the cuffs must remain extended over the hands.

(7) Tie back gowns may be fastened by the circulating practitioner.

(8) Wrap around gowns can be fastened with the assistance of other scrubbed team members or by the use of a sterile forcep. (National Association of Theatre Nurses, 2004)

GLOVING PROCEDURE

Gloves can be donned in the operating department by either a closed or an open method. Whichever method is used, it is important to minimise the risk of contamination from bare skin.

Closed method

(1) The circulating person opens the outside wrapper of the sterile glove pack and either offers this to the scrubbed member of staff or drops the inner pack onto a sterile field.

(2) Keeping the hands inside the gown cuffs, the sterile glove pack is opened so that the fingers are pointed towards the scrubbed member of staff.

(3) The first glove is picked up and positioned so that the palm of the glove is resting against the palm of the hand, with fingers pointing towards elbow and thumb against the wrist.

(4) Use the opposite hand (still inside the gown cuff) to pull the glove cuff over the outside of the gown cuff and over the back of the hand.
(5) Pull the glove cuff down to completely cover the gown cuff, positioning fingers and thumb comfortably inside the glove.
(6) Repeat with the other hand, using the already gloved fingers and thumb.

Open method

(1) The circulating person opens the outside wrapper of the sterile glove pack and drops the inner pack onto a sterile field.
(2) The inner glove pack is opened by the scrubbed practitioner so that the cuffs are pointing towards them.
(3) The first glove is picked up by the cuff, holding the inner surface only and taking care not to contaminate the outside surface of the glove.
(4) The glove is placed on the hand and pulled over the gown cuff, taking care that the bare hand only touches the inside of the sterile glove.
(5) The second glove is picked up using the fingers inside the fold between the glove and the cuff.
(6) Taking care not to touch the gloved hand with the bare hand, the glove is positioned and pulled over the second hand using the cuff.

PREVENTION OF SURGICAL SITE INFECTION
Surgical site infections account for up to 11% of infections acquired in hospitals (Emerson *et al.*, 1996). Surgical site infections can be:

- **Superficial** – involving the skin or subcutaneous tissue of the incision
- **Deep** – involving the fascial and muscle layers of the incision
- **Organ/space** – involving other areas than the incision opened or manipulated during the procedure

Surgical site infections are generally endogenous, that is acquired from the patient's own body bacteria:

- **Skin** – staphylococci and streptococci
- **Oral cavity and nasopharynx** – staphylococci, streptococci and anaerobic bacteria
- **Large bowel** – Gram negative bacilli and enterococci

Sources of surgical wound contamination include:

- Direct inoculation from the patient's own micro-organisms, from the surgeon's hands, from contaminated instruments or dressings, or from a break in sterile technique during a procedure
- Airborne contamination from the skin and clothing of staff and patients, or airflows in the operating theatre or ward
- Haematogenous spread via the bloodstream from infections at other body sites

The following practices and procedures should be applied to prevent surgical wound infection:

- Any obvious infections should be treated before planned and elective surgery.
- Hair should only be removed from the operation site if it will interfere with surgery. Shaving should not be used to remove hair; either clippers or a depilatory cream should be used. Hair removal should take place as near to the point of operation as possible.
- Prophylactic antibiotics should be administered at the appropriate times where prescribed.
- Blood glucose should be adequately controlled before and during surgery.
- The patient's body temperature should be maintained at normal during surgery, unless otherwise indicated, for example cardiac surgery.
- Pre-operative showering or bathing in an antiseptic, for example chlorhexidine gluconate, may be beneficial.
- An alcoholic skin preparation agent should be used to prepare the incision site. This should be applied in concentric circles moving outwards. Care should be taken to allow alcoholic

solutions to dry, particularly before use of a diathermy (Medical Devices Agency, 2000).

• Skin preparation solutions should be single use wherever possible. Where multi-use bottles are used they should not be refilled and should be used within the timeframe recommended by the manufacturer.

• A sterile wound dressing should be applied before the patient leaves the operating theatre.

• Closed system wound drainage should be used wherever possible. (Mangram *et al.*, 1999; Woodhead *et al.*, 2002; Department of Health, 2005)

POST-ANAESTHESIA CARE SETTINGS

The post-anaesthesia care unit comprises aspects of critical care areas, wards and the operating room. For example, as many patients are now transferred from the operating theatre to the post-anaesthesia care unit on their beds, the design of the unit should be such to allow appropriate physical space separation between beds to reduce risk of infection spread. In addition, units that are designated to provide intensive care support on a short-term basis should be designed to accommodate the infection prevention aspects important in intensive care units, for example adequate hand hygiene provision. Standard infection prevention principles (Chapter 5) apply to care and management of the patient in the post-anaesthesia care unit. For patients who require high dependency or intensive care level of management, the principles outlined in Chapter 13 apply.

MANAGEMENT OF SPECIFIC INFECTIONS IN THE PERI-OPERATIVE DEPARTMENT

Meticillin resistant Staphylococcus aureus and other multi-resistant bacteria

• The clinical team caring for the patient should ensure that the operating theatre is informed in advance of the patient's MRSA status in order for the correct precautions to be taken and the appropriate antibiotic prophylaxis given.

- Patients with MRSA need not be placed last on the operating list. However, a risk assessment should be undertaken and patients who are more likely to be heavily shedding MRSA, for example those with exfoliative skin conditions, may need to be placed last on the list.
- Good hand hygiene is imperative.
- Gloves and aprons should be worn by all peri-operative staff having direct contact with the patient.
- Patient contact surfaces should be cleaned or disinfected.
- To minimise the risk of airborne transmission of MRSA, conventionally ventilated operating theatres may be left empty for 15 minutes and ultraclean ventilated theatres for five minutes after a known MRSA case.
- Patients may be recovered in the post-anaesthesia care unit; however, it is sensible to allocate one member of staff to care for the patient. (National Association of Theatre Nurses, 2004; Coia *et al.*, 2006)

Infectious tuberculosis – patients with suspected or confirmed pulmonary tuberculosis whose sputum is positive for acid fast bacilli

- The clinical team caring for the patient should ensure that the operating theatre is informed in advance of the patient's tuberculosis status in order for the correct precautions to be taken.
- Infectious tuberculosis patients should be placed last on the operating list unless clinical need dictates otherwise.
- Patients must be brought to theatre immediately prior to surgery and must not wait in communal areas.
- A surgical mask should be worn by the patient during transfer.
- Disposable ventilation and respiratory equipment must be used.
- Anaesthetic and recovery staff must wear a high particulate filtration mask (FFP2 minimum).
- Gloves and aprons must be worn for close patient contact.
- Specimens must be labelled with a biohazard label.
- The patient should be recovered in the operating theatre or anaesthetic room and not the post-anaesthesia care unit.

- Patients should be transferred directly back to their single room.
- A theatre mask should be worn by the patient if clinical condition allows.
- Patient contact surfaces should be cleaned with detergent and water.
- Conventionally ventilated operating theatres should not be used for 15 minutes, ultraclean ventilated theatres for five minutes after a known infectious tuberculosis case. (The Interdepartmental Working Group on Tuberculosis, 1996)

Potentially infectious tuberculosis (patients whose sputum does not contain acid fast bacilli but in whom one or more cultures are positive) and closed tuberculosis (non-pulmonary tuberculosis e.g. kidney)

- The clinical team caring for the patient should ensure that the operating theatre is informed in advance of the patient's tuberculosis status in order for the correct precautions to be taken.
- Disposable ventilation and respiratory equipment must be used.
- Anaesthetic and recovery staff must wear a high particulate filtration mask (FFP2).
- Gloves and aprons must be worn for close patient contact.
- Specimens must be labelled with a biohazard label.
- Patient contact surfaces should be cleaned with detergent and water. (The Interdepartmental Working Group on Tuberculosis, 1996)

Patients with infective diarrhoea (e.g. *Clostridium difficile* or viral gastroenteritis)

- The clinical team caring for the patient should ensure that the operating theatre is informed in advance of the patient's infectious status in order for the correct precautions to be taken.
- Patients with diarrhoea/vomiting should only be brought to the operating theatre if there is an overriding clinical need.
- Staff should wear gloves and aprons for direct patient contact.

- Patient contact surfaces should be cleaned or disinfected.
- It is not necessary to leave the theatre empty for any period of time before the next case.
- Patients may be recovered in the post-anaesthesia care unit; however, it is sensible to allocate one member of staff to care for the patient.

Transmissible spongiform encephalopathies

Transmissible spongiform encephalopathies (TSEs) are fatal degenerative brain diseases that are found in both humans and animals. They are characterised by microscopic holes in the grey matter of the brain and in laboratory settings have been found to be transmissible by mouth and by percutaneous inoculation. TSEs include Creutzfeldt-Jakob disease (CJD), variant CJD (vCJD), Gerstmann Straussler-Scheinker syndrome, fatal familial insomnia and Kuru. All patients undergoing surgery should be assessed in advance to determine their risk of having a TSE as additional theatre and instrument decontamination procedures may be required. The risk assessment should determine whether the patient is symptomatic or in an at-risk category for CJD or vCJD. The following should be determined of all patients pre-operatively (Advisory Committee on Dangerous Pathogens and the Spongiform Encephalopathy Advisory Committee, 2003):

- Is there any history of CJD or other prion disease?
- Has the patient received growth hormone or gonadotropin therapy derived from human pituitary glands?
- Has the patient had brain or spinal cord surgery that included a dura mater graft?
- Has the patient been contacted as being at risk of vCJD or CJD for public health purposes?

The following theatre procedures apply to patients where the risk assessment has assessed them as symptomatic (definite, probable or possible CJD or vCJD):

- Place the patient last on the operating list to allow normal cleaning before the next theatre session.
- The minimum number of healthcare personnel should be involved in the procedure.

- Single use protective clothing must be worn and discarded after use as follows:

  — Liquid repellent operating gown over a plastic apron
  — Gloves
  — Mask and goggles or full face visor

- Use single use surgical items wherever possible. For reusable surgical items details on reprocessing are given below. (Advisory Committee on Dangerous Pathogens and the Spongiform Encephalopathy Advisory Committee, 2003)

For patients who are asymptomatic, but at risk of familial or iatrogenic CJD, the above precautions apply but protective clothing that is reusable may be used and processed by standard methods.

Table 12.2 details the requirements for decontamination of surgical instruments.

Table 12.2 Guidance on management of surgical instruments and CJD or vCJD.

Tissue infectivity	Status of patient			
CJD	**Definite/probable**	**Possible**	**At risk genetic**	**At risk iatrogenic**
High	Incinerate	Quarantine	Incinerate	Incinerate
Medium	Incinerate	Quarantine	Incinerate	Incinerate
Low	No special precautions	No special precautions	No special precautions	No special precautions
vCJD	**Definite/probable**	**Possible**		**At risk iatrogenic**
High	Incinerate	Quarantine		Incinerate
Medium	Incinerate	Quarantine		Incinerate
Low	No special precautions	No special precautions		No special precautions

Quarantining of instruments

Instruments that require quarantining for CJD or vCJD should be handled and stored safely. The following procedures should be observed:

- The appropriate protective clothing should be worn when directly handling the instruments (e.g. fluid repellent gown, gloves, eye and mouth protection).
- Using a sink in which water is continuously running, carefully hand wash the instruments, fully immersing them under the water, taking care not to create aerosols.
- Allow to air dry on a disposable instrument tray.
- When dry, place in an impervious rigid plastic container with a close fitting lid.
- Seal lid with heavy duty tape (e.g. autoclave tape).
- Label the box with patient details, surgical procedure details and the name of the responsible person (e.g. theatre sister).
- Store the sealed box in a suitable designated place. (Advisory Committee on Dangerous Pathogens and the Spongiform Encephalopathy Advisory Committee 2003)

SCENARIO

Miss Jones is a 32-year-old lady who is known to be a carrier of hepatitis C. She is due to have varicose vein surgery as a day case. What infection control precautions are required?

As for all surgical patients, Miss Jones' risk for CJD and vCJD should be assessed. The fact that Miss Jones has hepatitis C does not warrant any additional infection control precautions. Face protection, gowning and double gloving should be the same as would be applied to any patient undergoing varicose vein surgery.

SUMMARY

Infection prevention practices in the peri-operative setting aim to reduce the risk of blood borne viruses to staff and the risk of infection to patients from invasive procedures and surgical incisions. Standard infection control principles apply in this setting, with additional precautions to reduce exposure to blood.

REFERENCES

Advisory Committee on Dangerous Pathogens and the Spongiform Encephalopathy Advisory Committee (2003) *Transmissible Spongiform Encephalopathy Agents: Safe Working and the Prevention of Infection*. Available at: http://www.advisorybodies.doh.gov.uk/acdp/tseguidance/Index.htm (accessed 25 November 2006).

Association of Anaesthetists of Great Britain and Ireland (2002) *Infection Control in Anaesthesia*. Available at: http://www.aagbi.org/publications/guidelines/docs/infection02.pdf (accessed 25 November 2006).

Coia, J.E., Duckworth, G.K., Edwards, D.I., *et al.* (2006) Guidelines for the control and prevention of meticillin resistant *Staphylococcus aureus* (MRSA) in healthcare facilities. *Journal of Hospital Infection*, **63** (suppl.), s1–44.

Dawson, S.J. (2001) Epidural catheter infections. *Journal of Hospital Infection*, **47**, 3–8.

Department of Health (2005) *High Impact Intervention No. 3: Preventing Surgical Site Infection*. Available at: http://www.dh.gov.uk/assetRoot/04/11/34/74/04113474.pdf (accessed 25 November 2006).

Emmerson, A.M., Enstone, J.E., Griffin, M., Kelsey, M.C. and Smyth, E.T.M. (1996) The second national prevalence survey of infection in hospitals – overview of the results. *Journal of Hospital Infection*, **32** (3), 175–190.

European Standard EN 13795-1 (2002) *Surgical Drapes, Gowns and Clean Air Suits, Used as Medical Devices, for Patients, Clinical Staff and Equipment – Part 1: General Requirements for Manufacturers, Processors and Products*. British Standards Institution, London.

Holt, H.M., Andersen, S.S., Andersen, O., Gahrn-Hansen, B. and Siboni, K. (1995) Infections following epidural catheterisation. *Journal of Hospital Infection*, **30**, 253–260.

Mangram, A.J., Horan, T.C., Pearson, M.L., Silver, L.C., Jarvis, W.R., the Hospital Infection Control Practices Advisory Committee (1999) Guideline for prevention of surgical site infection, 1999. *Infection Control and Hospital Epidemiology*, **20** (4), 247–278.

Medical Devices Agency (2000) *Use of Spirit-based Solutions During Surgical Procedures Requiring the Use of Electosurgical Equipment SN 2000(17)*. Medical Devices Agency, London.

Multidisciplinary Working Group (2003) *Considering the Consequences: an Evaluation of Infection Risk when Choosing Surgical Gowns and Drapes in Today's NHS*. HSD Comunications, Rickmansworth.

National Association of Theatre Nurses (2004) *NATN Standards and Recommendations for Safe Perioperative Practice*. National Association of Theatre Nurses, Harrogate.

Ngan Kee, W.D., Jones, M.R., Thomas, P. and Worth, R.J. (1992) Extradural abscess complication following extradural anaesthesia for caesarean section. *British Journal of Anaesthesia*, **69**, 647–652.

Royal College of Nursing (2005) *Standards for Infusion Therapy*. Royal College of Nursing, London.

The Interdepartmental Working Group on Tuberculosis (1996) *The Prevention and Control of Tuberculosis in the United Kingdom: Recommendations for the Prevention and Control of Tuberculosis at Local Level.* Department of Health, London.

United Kingdom Health Departments (1998) *Guidance for Clinical Healthcare Workers: Protection Against Infection with Blood Borne Viruses.* The Stationery Office, London.

Woodhead, K., Taylor, E.W., Bannister, G., Chesworth, T., Hoffman, P. and Humphreys, H. (2002) Behaviours and rituals in the operating theatre: a report of the Hospital Infection Society Working Party on infection control in operating theatres. *Journal of Hospital Infection*, **51**, 241–255.

Specialist Care Settings 13

INTRODUCTION
Specialist care settings can have specific infection control requirements due to the types of organisms that cause infections. In
addition, patients' conditions and treatments can increase their
risk of acquiring an infection. This chapter covers the prevention
of infection in units where risk of infection is increased.

LEARNING OBJECTIVES
By the end of this chapter you will be able to:

❏ Discuss the specific hospital infection issues
❏ Describe infection prevention and control measures that apply
to:

— Intensive care units
— Cardiothoracic units
— Burn units
— Renal units

INTENSIVE CARE UNITS
Between 10 and 40% of patients admitted to an intensive care unit
develop an infection, with the commonest being pneumonia, followed by lower respiratory tract infection, urinary tract infection,
bacteraemia and wound infection (Humphreys *et al.*, 2000).
Patients in an intensive care unit are susceptible to infection due
to the range and extent of invasive procedures and monitoring
they will undergo, together with the immunosuppressive effects
of their underlying conditions. Standard infection control precautions apply in intensive care settings, but as a large proportion of
infections are pneumonia associated with ventilation, it is important to take all precautions possible to prevent infection.

PREVENTION OF VENTILATOR ASSOCIATED PNEUMONIA

Ventilator associated pneumonia (VAP) may account for up to 60% of all deaths linked to hospital infections (Tablan *et al.*, 2003). Where the VAP is due to *Pseudomonas* spp. or *Acinetobacter* spp. the mortality rate can be up to 73%. The following micro-organisms have been found to cause VAP:

- *Escherichia coli*
- *Klebsiella* spp.
- *Proteus* spp.
- *Streptococcus pneumoniae*
- *Haemophilus influenzae*
- *Pseudomonas aeruginosa*
- *Acinetobacter* spp.
- *Staphylococcus aureus* both meticillin sensitive and resistant

Infection occurs from aspiration of micro-organisms in the oral pharynx, haematogenous spread from infected cannulae sites or from right-sided endocarditis, or from exogenous sources. Hands are an important route of cross contamination during suctioning, manipulation of the tube and manipulation of the breathing circuit. Another route can be contaminated devices such as circuits, humidifiers and in-line nebulisers.

The following preventative measures should be applied to all ventilated patients to reduce the risk of VAP (Berenholtz *et al.*, 2002; Fullbrook and Mooney, 2003; Tablan *et al.*, 2003; Department of Health, 2005).

Preventing aspiration

- Use non-invasive methods of ventilation wherever possible.
- Avoid repeat endotracheal intubation.
- Use orotracheal as opposed to nasotracheal intubation.
- Position the head of the bed at an angle of 30–45°.
- Clear secretions from around the cuff before deflating.

Preventing complications of critical care

- Give prophylaxis to prevent deep vein thrombosis.
- Give prophylaxis to prevent gastric ulceration.

- Reduce duration of mechanical ventilation using sedation holding.

Infection prevention practices

- Decontaminate hands before and after any manipulation of the breathing circuit, equipment and intubation tube.
- Wear gloves in accordance with standard precautions, donning a fresh pair of gloves before handling of the breathing circuit and intubation tube. If non-sterile gloves are being used these should have been obtained from a clean glove box immediately before use and not from one located in a dirty utility area.
- Wear apron and face protection in accordance with standard precautions.

Care of equipment

- Thoroughly clean all respiratory equipment before disinfection or sterilisation.
- Use steam sterilisation or high level disinfection (see Chapter 16) for reprocessing of respiratory devices.
- Sterile water should be used for rinsing when cleaning or disinfecting respiratory devices.
- Single use respiratory devices should not be decontaminated against manufacturers' advice.
- Do not routinely change breathing circuits with humidifiers. They should only be changed if visibly soiled or malfunctioning.
- Do not allow condensate in the tubing to drain towards the patient.
- Periodically drain and discard the condensate into a single use or disinfected receptacle.
- Only sterile water should be used for humidification.
- Do not routinely change heat moisture exchangers more often than every 48 hours unless visibly soiled or malfunctioning.
- Do not routinely change breathing circuits attached to a heat moisture exchanger.
- Follow manufacturers' instructions for use and changing of oxygen humidifiers.

- For small volume nebulisers, decontaminate between use on the same patient, using sterile water for washing and rinsing.
- Only use sterile nebulisation fluid from a single dose vial.

Suctioning

- Wear protective clothing in accordance with standard precautions (gloves, apron, goggles).
- Decontaminate hands before and after carrying out suction procedures.
- If closed system suctioning is used, change in accordance with manufacturers' instructions.
- Use a sterile single use catheter for open suctioning.
- Use sterile fluid to remove secretions from the catheter if it is to be used to re-enter the lower respiratory tract. (Day *et al.*, 2002; Moore, 2003; Dougherty and Lister, 2004)

Infection prevention in management of tracheostomies

- Cannula dressing should be performed using an aseptic technique.
- Hands should be decontaminated before handling any component of the tracheostomy.
- Suction should be carried out using a clean technique.
- If the tracheostomy has a reusable inner tube it should be decontaminated in accordance with manufacturers' instructions and stored in a manner that protects it from contamination. (McConnell, 2002; Dougherty and Lister, 2004; Lewis and Oliver, 2005)

CARDIOTHORACIC UNITS

Prevention of infection associated with pacemaker devices
Infection associated with cardiac pacemaker implantation can be as high as 19% (Victor *et al.*, 1999). Whilst this may be confined locally to the subcutaneous 'pocket' in which the pacemaker generator is sited, infection of the implanted electrodes and endocarditis can occur (Voet *et al.*, 1999) and can be life threatening. Staphylococci are the most common causative micro-organisms,

with *Staphylococcus aureus* causing early infection and *Staphylococcus epidermidis* more commonly associated with late infection (Klug *et al.*, 1997). Risk factors for infection include:

- Repeated surgical procedures related to the pacemaker pocket
- Post-insertion haemorrhage or necrosis
- Patients with diabetes mellitus
- Older patients
- Patients with intravenous catheters already in situ

To prevent infection, principles for prevention of surgical site infection should be followed (see Chapter 12) together with these following specific principles:

- The pacemaker should be implanted in a facility with air quality of theatre standard wherever possible.
- The minimum number of personnel required to carry out the procedure should be present.
- Implantation should be carried out using as sterile a technique as possible.
- Good surgical haemostasis should be assured.
- Prophylactic antibiotics may be given.
- Temporary pacing should be avoided, but if necessary it should be used for the shortest time possible. (Voet *et al.*, 1999)

Following implantation of the pacemaker, the surgical wound should be managed in accordance with all types of wound healing by primary intention in that:

- The dressing should be left in situ and not removed unless essential in the initial post-operative period.
- An aseptic procedure should be used for dressing changes or manipulations.

Temporary pacing systems have a higher risk of infection, as the point at which the leads exit the skin provides an access point for micro-organisms that allows direct access to the bloodstream. Up to 20% of patients with temporary pacing wires develop bacteraemia if the wires are left in for longer than 48 hours (Murphy, 2001). Pacing wire exit points should be covered with a sterile dressing to protect them from micro-organisms in the environment and should only be exposed when absolutely necessary. An aseptic technique should be used when handling the wires as they exit the skin. Any dressing procedures should be carried out aseptically. Temporary pacing wires should be removed at the earliest opportunity.

Management of chest drains

Chest drains are inserted to relieve a pneumothorax, to drain malignant pleural effusions and empyema, to treat traumatic hae-mopneumothorax or post-cardiac and thoracic surgery. Infection rates for drains inserted due to trauma may be as high as 12% (Fallon and Wears, 1992). Chest drains should be inserted using an aseptic technique (Laws *et al.*, 2003), with prophylactic antibiotics considered for those inserted in trauma patients. Chest drains are connected to a single flow drainage system, for example an underwater sealed drain, therefore limiting the risk of infection arising via the lumen of the tube. Water used to fill underwater drain bottles must be sterile at the point of use and care should be taken to prevent contamination during filling and emptying of drain bottles. The drain exit site should be covered with a sterile dressing, preferably a film dressing to allow visual checks of the exit site.

BURN UNITS

Burns patients are susceptible to infection because one of the primary barriers to infection, the skin, is breached (Lederer *et al.*, 1999). Infection is the leading cause of mortality in patients in a burn unit, with up to 55% developing a hospital acquired infection; it is also not uncommon for burns patients to suffer more than one infection during their hospital stay (Santucci *et al.*, 2003). Both Gram negative and Gram positive organisms are responsible for these infections, with *Staphylococcus aureus*, *Pseudomonas aeruginosa*, *Acinetobacter* spp. and coagulase negative staphylococci being the commonest causes of infection. Infection in burns patients is not confined to the burns wound itself but, due to the critical nature of care, pneumonia, bloodstream and urinary tract infections are common in this patient group. Burns patients acquire organisms from their own microbial flora (endogenous) and from the hospital care and environment (exogenous). Burns wounds initially become colonised with Gram positive micro-organisms, but over time these are replaced by Gram negative micro-organisms and if the burn wound is exposed for long periods of time, antibiotic resistant organisms and fungi can be found in burns patients. Gram negative micro-organisms are 50% more likely to cause mortality in burns patients than Gram positive micro-organisms (Mason *et al.*, 1986). Burns patients are also susceptible to infection from antibiotic resistant micro-organisms. Outbreaks of MRSA (meticillin resistant *Staphylococcus aureus*) have occurred in burn units; therefore, infection prevention strategies must include factors that prevent these and other antibiotic organisms.

Prevention of infection in burns patients requires an integrated approach that ensures patients are cared for in an appropriate environment and with the highest standard of clinical care. The environment for patients with burns will vary depending on whether the healthcare facility is classified as a burn facility, burn centre or burn unit, with the complexity of the care required determining in which type of facility a patient should be managed (National Burn Care Review Committee, undated). However, the basic principles for providing a safe, clean environment will apply regardless of the grading of a burn facility. For burn facilities, single room accommodation should be available but not all the beds need to be in single rooms. For burn units single room accommodation for the beds is recommended, with close access to an operating theatre. Burn centres require single room accommodation that has air filtration and temperature regulation. The single rooms should be at positive pressure to the corridor air to avoid airborne micro-organisms from the outside entering a patient's room. An operating theatre, which is dedicated to burn care, should be attached to the patient accommodation.

Compliance with good hand hygiene is vital in burn facilities. Due to the increased susceptibility of patients to infection, and the increased risk of antibiotic resistant micro-organisms, an antiseptic solution should be considered for hand washing. Protective clothing in the form of gloves and aprons should be worn in accordance with standard precautions, but with the knowledge that contact with large numbers of micro-organisms is likely in burn injured patients. Non-essential equipment should not be kept in patients' rooms and in the care of children soft toys should be avoided unless they can be adequately laundered regularly. Other non-essential items should be avoided, including plants, flowers and cards. Clinical equipment should be dedicated to individual patients or adequately decontaminated between use (see Chapter 16). When determining the decontamination process it is important to be aware of the increased possibility of contact with non-intact skin due to the skin loss associated with the burn injury. Hydrotherapy has been associated with outbreaks of *Acinetobacter baumanii* (Simor *et al.*, 2002), *Pseudomonas aeruginosa* (Richard *et al.*, 1994) and MRSA (Rutala *et al.*, 1983). Hydrotherapy should be avoided whilst burns patients have extensive areas of skin that cannot be completely covered by a waterproof dressing. All dressings should be undertaken using an aseptic technique (see Chapter 10). However, additional infection prevention considerations may be needed, for example sterile quality outer bandages (Christiaens *et al.*, 2005).

RENAL UNITS

Renal units have specific infection control needs due to the extensive contact that staff are likely to have with blood, as well as patient factors that increase their risk of infection, including the use of immunosuppressive therapy for transplant recipients and invasive devices for dialysis.

Prevention of blood borne viruses

Both staff and patients have acquired hepatitis B in renal dialysis units (Knight *et al.*, 1970), and more recently hepatitis C has been transmitted between patients on a renal unit (Allander *et al.*, 1994). Human immunodeficiency virus (HIV) transmission has also been reported (Velandia *et al.*, 1995). Transmission of blood borne viruses from patient to patient has been associated with the use of multiple dose vials, blood transfusions, contaminated dialysis equipment, environmental surfaces and reprocessing of dialysers and dialysis needles. Standard infection control principles (see Chapter 5) should be implemented in dialysis units, with the following enhanced prevention measures:

- Patients on dialysis or in immunisation programmes should be vaccinated against hepatitis B.
- Staff in renal units who have clinical contact with patients should be immunised against hepatitis B.
- A programme for testing patients for blood borne viruses in certain circumstances, for example after dialysing abroad, should be in place.
- Strict adherence to standard precautions should be in place at all times.
- Relatives and friends who assist in dialysis procedures should be trained in blood borne virus prevention measures and offered vaccination against hepatitis B.
- Patients with blood borne viruses should receive dialysis in an area segregated from the main dialysis unit.
- Staff should be designated to care for a patient with a blood borne virus alone and should not care for other dialysis patients at the same time.
- Separate dialysis machines must be used for patients infected with hepatitis B.
- For patients infected with hepatitis C and HIV a separate dialysis machine is not needed but machines must be cleaned and disinfected in accordance with manufacturers' instructions between use.
- Single use blood tubing sets must be discarded after a single dialysis session on one patient.
- If there is evidence that the filter on the venous pressure monitoring line has had contact with blood then this should be replaced.
- Rupture of this filter requires that all potentially contaminated machine components be adequately decontaminated or replaced.
- Dialysis fluid circuits should be decontaminated between use in accordance with manufacturers' instructions.
- External surfaces of dialysis machines should be disinfected daily and after use on a patient with a blood borne virus. A chlorine based disinfectant at 1000 ppm should be used.
- Single use dialysers should be discarded after use.

- Staff who have skin conditions where there are extensive areas of non-intact skin (e.g. eczema) should not work in dialysis units.
- Staff should be supervised until deemed competent in safe working practices to prevent blood borne virus transmission.
- Bed spacing in dialysis units should be sufficient to allow safe working practices.
- Protective clothing should be available at the point of patient care.
- Sharps containers should be located at the point of patient care.
- Multi-use vials should be designated to individual patients.
- Staff should not eat or drink on the unit unless in designated rest areas.
- Patients should have their bed location and the dialysis machine used logged at each session in event of an outbreak 'look-back' exercise. (Centers for Disease Control and Prevention, 2001; Department of Health, 2002)

Prevention of infection associated with dialysis access

Central venous catheters are used as a temporary access for hae-modialysis but these devices have an associated risk of bacterae-mia (George *et al.*, 2006). Femoral catheters have a high risk of infection and should, therefore, only be used as a temporary access for up to one week (National Kidney Foundation, 2000). The preferred method of venous access for haemodialysis is an arteriovenous fistula (Renal Association, 2002). The risk of bacte-raemia in renal patients with a central venous catheter is at least seven times greater than with an arteriovenous fistula (Hoen *et al.*, 1998). Patients in renal units are more susceptible to antibi-otic resistant micro-organisms, including MRSA and vancomycin resistant enterococci (VRE) (Grabsch *et al.*, 2006). These micro-organisms are common causes of infection associated with central venous access devices; therefore, renal dialysis units and other areas where haemodialysis takes place (e.g. intensive care units) should ensure policies and practices are in place to reduce spread of these micro-organisms. In addition to the general principles for insertion and management of central venous lines, as described in Chapter 8, the following care principles should be applied to haemodialysis lines:

- The line should be inserted in a clean environment.
- Only staff who are trained and competent should access or handle the line.
- An aseptic technique must be used for all handling of the line.
- A dry gauze dressing is recommended by the Renal Association in preference to transparent dressings.
- The hub of the dialysis line should be disinfected (e.g. with chlorhexidine gluconate in alcohol before accessing the line). (Renal Association, 2006)

To prevent bacteraemias associated with accessing arteriovenous fistulas the following principles should be applied:

- An aseptic technique should be used for all access procedures (i.e. hand hygiene and use of gloves).
- The site for access should be located and palpated before any skin preparation technique.
- The access site should be washed with an antibacterial soap and water.
- The access site should be cleaned with an alcoholic antiseptic solution (e.g. chlorhexidine or povidone iodine), in a circular motion, allowing time for the alcohol to dry before inserting the dialysis needle.
- A non-touch technique should be used for needle insertion.
- If gloves are contaminated during the cannulation procedure they should be changed. (Jindal et al., 1999)

Prevention of infection associated with peritoneal dialysis

Peritoneal dialysis (PD) involves the administration, retention and then release of a dialysis fluid into the abdominal cavity, using the peritoneal membrane to filter out waste products that are not being removed due to renal failure. A permanent peritoneal dialysis catheter is inserted into the patient's abdomen by surgical procedure. Infectious complications associated with PD include catheter exit site infections, tunnel infections and peritonitis. Peritonitis has been reported in up to 20% of patients undergoing peritoneal dialysis (Hasbargen et al., 1993). Exit site infection is characterised by redness, inflammation and purulent discharge at the catheter site, and peritonitis is characterised by abdominal pain or distension, fever and cloudy dialysis fluid (Swartz, 1999). PD associated infections can be caused by a variety of micro-organisms, including *Staphylococcus aureus*, coagulase negative staphylococci, *Streptococcus* spp. and *Enterococcus* spp.

To prevent infections associated with peritoneal dialysis the following principles should be applied:

- Prophylactic antibiotics should be considered when PD catheters are being inserted.
- Mupirocin ointment applied to the exit site in the immediate post-insertion period is recommended in some care protocols.
- An aseptic technique should be used for exit site care in the initial post-insertion period; once the exit site is healed, a clean technique can be used.
- The exit site should be kept dry until healed.
- The exit site should be redressed when wet and after bathing.
- 'Flush before fill' dialysis systems should be used in preference, to prevent risk of contamination during spiking. (Joanna Briggs Institute, 2004; Piraino *et al.*, 2005)

SCENARIO

Mr Walker is a 36-year-old man who is in the intensive care unit following a road traffic accident that has resulted in major trauma to his head and lower limbs. He is currently ventilated and is in acute renal failure. He is being dialysed through a temporary dialysis line. What are the important care management principles that should be in place to reduce his risk of infection?

Mr Walker is at risk of ventilator associated pneumonia. He should be nursed with the head of his bed at an angle of 30–45°; prophylaxis should be given to prevent deep vein thrombosis and gastric ulceration. Mechanical ventilation should be stopped as soon as his condition allows. The temporary dialysis line should only be handled by competent staff. An aseptic technique should be used for all handling of the line. Unnecessary access to the dialysis line should be avoided.

SUMMARY

Patients in specialist care units are at increased risk of infection due to the nature of their conditions and the associated treatments. The use of invasive devices is commonplace in specialist care units, where the adoption of aseptic techniques for handling of these devices is an essential component of infection prevention.

REFERENCES

Allander, T., Medin, C., Jacobson, S.H., Grillner, L. and Persson, M.A.A. (1994) Hepatitis C transmission in a haemodialysis unit: molecular evidence for spread of virus among patients not sharing equipment. *Journal of Medical Virology*, **43**, 415–419.

Berenholtz, S.M., Dorman, T. and Ngo, K. (2002) Qualitative review of intensive care unit quality indicators. *Journal of Critical Care*, **17**, 12–15.

Centers for Disease Control and Prevention (2001) Recommendations for preventing transmission of infection among chronic haemodialysis patients. *Morbidity and Mortality Weekly Report*, **50**, 1–43.

Christiaens, G., Hayette, M.P., Jacquemin, D., Melin, P., Mutsers, J. and De Mol, P. (2005) An outbreak of *Absidia carymbifera* infection associated with bandage contamination in a burn unit. *Journal of Hospital Infection*, **61** (1), 88.

Day, T., Farnell, S., Haynes, S., Wainwright, S. and Wilson-Barnett, J. (2002) Tracheal suctioning: an exploration of nurses' knowledge and competence in acute and high dependency ward areas. *Journal of Advanced Nursing*, **39** (1), 35–45.

Department of Health (2002) *Good Practice Guidelines for Renal Dialysis/Transplantation Units: Prevention and Control of Blood Borne Virus Infection*. Department of Health, London.

Department of Health (2005) *Saving Lives: a Delivery Programme to Reduce Healthcare Associated Infection Including MRSA*. Department of Health, London.

Dougherty, L. and Lister, S. (eds) (2004) *The Royal Marsden Hospital Manual of Clinical Nursing Procedures* (sixth edition). Blackwell Publishing, Oxford.

Fallon, W.F. and Wears, R.L. (1992) Prophylactic antibiotics for the prevention of infectious complications, including empyema, following tube thoracoscopy for trauma: results of a meta-analysis. *Journal of Trauma*, **33**, 110–117.

Fulbrook, P. and Mooney, S. (2003) Care bundles in critical care: a practical approach to evidence based practice. *Nursing in Critical Care*, **8** (6), 249–255.

George, A., Tokars, J.I., Clutterbuck, E.J., Bamford, K.B., Pusey, C. and Holmes, A.H. (2006) Reducing dialysis associated bacteraemia, and recommendations for surveillance in the United Kingdom: prospective study. *British Medical Journal*, **332** (7555), 1435.

Grabsch, E.A., Burrell, L.J., Padglione, A., O'Keeffe, J.M., Ballard, S. and Grayson, M.L. (2006) Risk of environmental and healthcare worker contamination with vancomycin resistant enterococci during outpatient procedures and hemodialysis. *Infection Control and Hospital Epidemiology*, **27** (3), 287–293.

Hasbargen, B.J., Rodgers, D.J., Hasbargen, J.A., Quinn, M.J. and James, M.K. (1993) Exit site care – is it time for a change? *Peritoneal Dialysis International*, **13**, s313–315.

Hoen, B., Paul-Dauphin, A., Hestin, D. and Kessler, M. (1998) EPI-BACDIAL: a multi-centre prospective study of risk factors for bacteraemia in chronic haemodialysis patients. *Journal of the American Society of Nephrologists*, **9**, 869–867.

Humphreys, H., Willats, S. and Vincent, J.L. (2000) *Intensive Care Infections*. W.B. Saunders, London.

Jindal, K.K., Ethier, J.H., Lindsay, R.M. *et al.* (1999) Clinical practice guidelines for vascular access. *Journal of the American Society of Nephrology*, 10, s287–321.

Joanna Briggs Institute (2004) Clinical effectiveness of different approaches to peritoneal dialysis catheter exit site care. *Best Practice*, **8** (1), 1–7.

Klug, D., Lacroix, D., Savoye, C. *et al.* (1997) Systemic infection related to endocarditis on pacemaker leads. *Circulation*, **95**, 2098–2107.

Knight, A.H., Fox, R.A., Baillod, R.A., Niazi, S.P., Sherlock, S. and Moorhead, J.F. (1970) Hepatitis associated antigen and antibody in haemodialysis patients and staff. *British Medical Journal*, **iii**, 603–606.

Laws, D., Neville, E. and Duffy, J. (2003) BTS guidelines for the insertion of a chest drain. *Thorax*, **58** (ii), 53.

Lederer, J.A., Rodrick, M.L. and Mannick, J.A. (1999) The effects of injury on the adaptive immune response. *Shock*, **11**, 153–159.

Lewis, T. and Oliver, G. (2005) Improving tracheostomy care for ward patients. *Nursing Standard*, **19** (19), 33–37.

McConnell, E. (2002) Providing tracheostomy care. *Nursing*, **January**, 17.

Mason Jr, A.D., McManus, A.T. and Pruitt Jr, B.A. (1986) Association of Burn Mortality and Bacteraemia: a 25-year review. *Archives of Surgery*, **121**, 1027–1031.

Moore, T. (2003) Suctioning techniques for the removal of respiratory secretions. *Nursing Standard*, **18** (9), 47–53.

Murphy, J.J. (2001) Problems with temporary cardiac pacing. *British Medical Journal*, **323**, 527.

National Burn Care Review Committee (undated) *Standards and Strategy for Burn Care: a Review of Burn Care in the British Isles*. National Burn Care Review Committee, London.

National Kidney Foundation (2000) Clinical practice guidelines for vascular access. *American Journal of Kidney Disease*, **37** (suppl. 1), 137–180.

Piraino, B., Bailie, G.R., Bernardini, J. *et al.* (2005) Peritoneal dialysis related infection recommendations: 2005 update. *Peritoneal Dialysis International*, **25**, 107–131.

Renal Association (2002) *Treatment of Adults and Children with Renal Failure: Standards and Audit Measures* (third edition*).* Renal Association, London.

Renal Association (2006) *Clinical Practice Guidelines: Guideline 3A Haemodialysis* (draft). Available at: http://www.renal.org/guidelines/module3a.html (accessed 20 November 2006).

Richard, P., Floch, R.L., Chamoux, C., Pannier, M., Espaze, E. and Richet, H. (1994) *Pseudomonas aeruginosa* outbreak in a burn unit: role of antimicrobials in the emergence of multiple resistant strains. *Journal of Infectious Diseases*, **170**, 377–383.

Rutala W.A., Katz, E.B., Sheretz, R.J. and Savubbi Jr, F.A. (1983) Environmental study of meticillin resistant *Staphylococcus aureus* epidemic in a burn unit. *Journal of Clinical Microbiology*, **18**, 683–688.

Santucci, S.G., Gobara, S., Santos, C.R., Fontana, C. and Levin, S. (2003) Infections in a burn intensive care unit: experience of seven years. *Journal of Hospital Infection*, **53**, 6–13.

Simor, A., Lee, M., Vearncombe, M. *et al.* (2002) An outbreak due to multi-resistant *Acinetobacter baumannii* in a burn unit: risk factors for acquisition and management. *Infection Control and Hospital Epidemiology*, **23**, 261–267.

Swartz, R.D. (1999) Exit site and catheter care: review of important issues. *Advances in Peritoneal Dialysis*, **15**, 201–204.

Tablan, O.C., Anderson, L.J., Besser, R., Bridges, C. and Hajjeh, R. (2003) *Guidelines for Preventing Healthcare Associated Pneumonia.* Available from: www.cdc.gov (accessed 20 November 2006).

Velandia, M., Fridkin, S.K., Cardenas, V. *et al.* (1995) Transmission of HIV in dialysis centre. *Lancet*, **345**, 1417–1422.

Victor, F., De Place, C., Camus, C. *et al.* (1999) Pacemaker lead infection: echocardiographic features, management and outcome. *Heart*, 81, 82–87.

Voet, J.G., Vanderkerckhove, Y.R., Muyldermans, L.L., Missault, L.H. and Matthys, L.J. (1999) Pacemaker lead infection: report of three cases and review of the literature. *Heart*, **81**, 88–91.

14 | The Isolated Patient

INTRODUCTION

In addition to standard infection control precautions, additional isolation precautions are sometimes required to prevent the spread of specific infections both from and to patients. Caring for patients in isolation requires not only an understanding and appreciation of infection control precautions, but awareness of the physical and psychological effects of segregation in isolation rooms. This chapter covers the assessment of need for isolation and the management of patients in isolation.

LEARNING OBJECTIVES

By the end of this chapter you will be able to:

❑ Describe the facilities required for patient isolation
❑ Discuss the key principles in caring for patients in source
❑ Discuss the psychological care of patients in isolation

THE NEED FOR ISOLATION

Standard precautions (as described in Chapter 5) are applied to the care of all patients in hospital. However, these will not prevent the spread of micro-organisms transmitted by the airborne route; nor are they always sufficient to prevent the spread of specific micro-organisms that are of importance in hospitals, for example multiple resistant bacteria. Isolation can also be used to prevent the spread of infection to patients who are particularly susceptible to hospital infection, for example neutropenic patients undergoing chemotherapy. Decisions on patient isolation are not always straightforward to make; an assessment must be made of the risk of infection to and from other patients in the vicinity as well as the patient's clinical and psychological condition. The questions to ask when making decisions in respect of isolation are:

- What is the micro-organism we are concerned about?
- What is the source of the micro-organism (for example is it found in respiratory secretions or urine)?
- How is it spread (airborne, contact, droplet, faecal-oral, or percutaneous)?
- What is the route of entry into another patient?

Other considerations are also taken into account (Gopal Rao and Jeanes, 1999) including:

- Whether there is evidence of person-to-person spread in hospitals
- Whether the bacteria have significant antibiotic resistance
- How prevalent is the micro-organism in the hospital:
  — Sporadic – only present occasionally
  — Endemic – often present
  — Epidemic – an outbreak situation
  — What is the risk of dispersal, for example if the micro-organisms are on the skin does the patient have eczema and is therefore more likely to be shedding large numbers into the environment?

Once the infection risk has been assessed, the other patient care risks should be considered, for example:

- Is the patient at risk of falling if placed in a single room?
- Is there a risk of the patient's clinical condition deteriorating if they cannot be constantly observed?
- Will the patient suffer significant psychological effects from isolation?

If the assessment of all risks indicates that the risks to the individual patient are at least as great or greater than the risk of infection to other patients and isolation of an infectious patient is not instituted, then adequate documentation of this assessment and decision should be undertaken and a plan or care management instituted that minimises risk of infection to other patients.

ISOLATION FACILITIES

One of the most important aspects of patient isolation is patient placement (Garner *et al.*, 1996). The design of isolation facilities varies from single rooms attached to wards to specialised isolation rooms in infectious disease facilities. Isolation rooms can be categorised as follows (NHS Estates, 2002).

Single room   a room with space for one patient and accompanying furniture, such as bed, locker, chair, table and a hand washing basin.

En suite single room   as above but with en suite facilities that may consist of toilet, shower and bath.

Isolation room   as above but with specialist ventilation so that the air inside is either at positive or negative pressure to the air outside. A lobby may or may not be included in the design (Figure 14.1). Negative pressure rooms are used for patients who

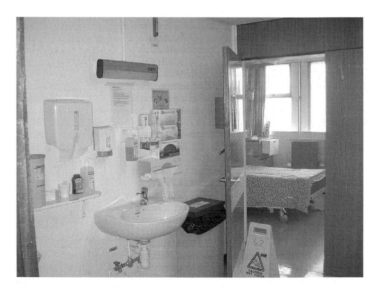

Figure 14.1 Isolation room with lobby.

are isolated because they are a risk of infection to other patients, for example patients with multi-drug resistant tuberculosis. When the door is opened the air from outside the room is sucked into the room by the negative pressure inside. Air from the room is generally exhausted to the outside via a filter and away from air inlets to other ward or department areas. Positive pressure rooms are used for patients who are at specific risk of infection from other patients and the outside clinical environment. Air that enters the room is filtered to remove particles and micro-organisms that could be harmful to immunocompromised patients. The air inside the room is kept at a higher pressure than that outside the room so that when the door is opened air from outside the room does not enter the room. Negative and positive pressure rooms are generally continually monitored to ensure the pressure remain as set using either a light system or a pressure gauge (Figures 14.2 and 14.3). It is important that ward staff check and record that air pressures in isolation rooms are sufficient on a regular basis.

FUNDAMENTALS OF ISOLATION PRECAUTIONS FOR THE INFECTED PATIENT

The following fundamental principles apply to isolation of patients (Garner *et al.*, 1996). Protective isolation for patients at risk of infection is covered in Chapter 15.

Patient placement

Following the assessment of risks, patients are placed into isolation facilities accordingly. Table 14.1 details suggested isolation facilities for infections commonly encountered in UK hospitals. The door must remain closed for all airborne infections. For infections spread by the contact route the door may be left open, but should be closed when carrying out activities that could lead to airborne dispersal of micro-organisms, for example bedmaking for patients with meticillin-resistant *Staphylococcus aureus* (MRSA). Whilst complying with patient confidentiality, there should be a means to identify to all staff and visitors that this is a room being used for isolation. Signs that indicate the precautions to be taken by staff and visitors are useful. An example of such a sign is given in Figure 14.4.

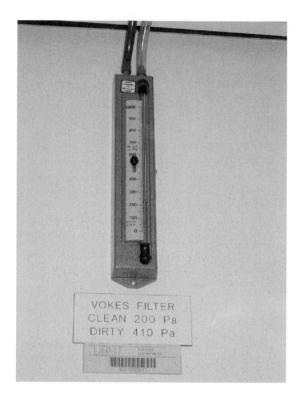

Figure 14.2 Gauge for monitoring isolation room pressures.

Hand hygiene

Hand decontamination should be performed before entering and when leaving a single or isolation room. This may be performed using alcohol gel, liquid soap or antiseptic soap, depending on the micro-organism or infection. Chapter 5 gives further detail on hand decontamination agents and their use.

Protective clothing

Gloves are worn when entering the room of an isolated patient to reduce the risk of healthcare workers' hands becoming contaminated with micro-organisms. Gloves should be removed on

Table 14.1 Patient placement for isolation.

Infection/micro-organism	Isolation placement
Clostridium difficile	Single room with en suite facilities
Campylobacter gastroenteritis	Single room with en suite facilities
Chickenpox (varicella zoster)	Single room
Vancomycin resistant enterococci	Single room
Escherichia coli 0157 diarrhoea	Single room with en suite facilities
Rotavirus gastroenteritis	Single room with en suite facilities
Salmonella	Single room with en suite facilities
Meticillin resistant *Staphylococcus aureus*	Single room with en suite facilities
Hepatitis A and E with diarrhoea	Single room with en suite facilities
Influenza	Single room with en suite facilities
Parainfluenza	Single room with en suite facilities
Avian influenza	Negative pressure isolation room
Measles	Single room with en suite facilities
Meningitis	Single room preferable
Mumps	Single room with en suite facilities
Norovirus	Single room with en suite facilities
Pertussis (whooping cough)	Single room if other vulnerable babies
Extended spectrum beta-lactamase producing Gram negatives (ESBLs)	Single room preferable
Respiratory syncytial virus	Single room
Rubella (German measles)	Single room with en suite facilities
Shigella gastroenteritis	Single room with en suite facilities
Streptococcal disease (group A)	Single room with en suite facilities in surgical, intensive care and obstetric settings
Tuberculosis (open/infectious)	Single room with en suite facilities
Multi-drug resistant tuberculosis	Negative pressure isolation room

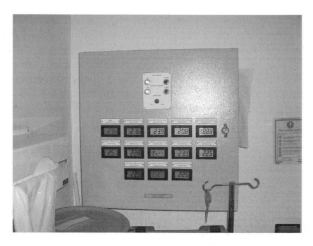

Figure 14.3 Light system for monitoring air pressure in isolation rooms.

ISOLATION PRECAUTIONS

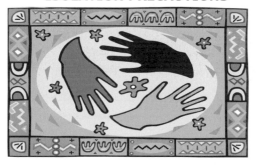

REPORT TO NURSE IN CHARGE BEFORE ENTERING

Figrue 14.4 Example isolation sign.

leaving the isolation room. If there is a need to continue wearing gloves on leaving the isolation room (for example when disposing of a urine bottle) the original pair of gloves should be removed and a clean pair donned. Gowns or aprons are worn to reduce the risk of healthcare workers' clothing becoming contaminated with micro-organisms. The gown/apron should be donned before entering the room and removed on leaving. Eye protection is worn in accordance with standard precautions (see Chapter 5). Masks are also worn in accordance with standard precautions. For some isolated patients, specific masks/respirators are required, for example patients with open/infectious tuberculosis. Masks are also discarded on leaving the isolation room. Gloves and aprons/gowns may need to be kept in the isolation/single room to enable staff to change these items when moving from a dirty to a clean task whilst in the room. To reduce risk of staff contaminating themselves whilst removing protective clothing it should be removed in the following order:

(1) Remove gloves, taking care not to contaminate hands in the process and discard as clinical waste.
(2) Remove eye protection (if worn) and discard as clinical waste if disposable, or place into the appropriate receptacle for decontamination if reusable.
(3) Remove mask, handling by the ties/elastic only, avoiding contact with the front of the mask, and discard as clinical waste.
(4) Remove apron/gown, breaking the plastic neck and/or back ties. Remove carefully, taking care not to contaminate clothing and discard as clinical waste.
(5) Decontaminate hands thoroughly.

Patient care equipment
Equipment used for care of the isolated patient should be dedicated to their use alone whilst they are in isolation, wherever possible. Examples of such equipment include manual handling aids, stethoscopes, commodes, monitoring equipment, drip stands, pumps. On removal from the single or isolation room these items must be adequately decontaminated before being stored or used on another patient. Chapter 16 gives detailed

guidance on equipment decontamination. Multiple patient equipment that is taken into single or isolation rooms must be decontaminated before use on another patient, for example blood pressure monitoring cuffs. Nursing and medical notes, drug and observation charts, and bedside folders should not be taken into the single/isolation room. All staff must have decontaminated their hands before handling these items.

Linen

Laundry should be bagged and handled in accordance with local policy. For patients in isolation there is often a requirement that linen be double bagged in red linen bags, with the inner liner bag being disposable (NHS Executive, 1995). The inner liner bag should be kept inside the single/isolation room. This should be sealed when two thirds full and placed into the outer bag on removal from the room.

Waste

Waste should be bagged and handled in accordance with local policy. This may mean that not all waste is classed as clinical waste and segregation may be needed (NHS Estates, 2004). Waste should be bagged inside the isolation/single room and the bags or bins closed/sealed on removal from the room. Double bagging of waste is not generally required, neither is segregation of waste from isolation/single rooms during collection and disposal procedures.

Cutlery and crockery

Disposable cutlery and crockery is generally not required for patients in single/isolation rooms. Hospital dishwashers use a combination of hot water and detergent to adequately decontaminate cutlery and crockery. Reusable cutlery and crockery should be washed in a dishwasher out of preference.

Cleaning

It is important that daily cleaning of single/isolation rooms takes place at a minimum in accordance with normal cleaning schedules. Additional cleaning may be needed, for example additional toilet cleaning for patients with infectious diarrhoea. Separate cleaning equipment is required for isolation/single rooms and this should be adequately decontaminated after use. Cleaning solutions are generally dictated by local policy but it is common to use a disinfectant, for example chlorine, for cleaning isolation/single rooms. When the isolated patient leaves the isolation/single room then an extensive clean is required. This is generally carried out using a disinfectant solution but local policy should be followed. The following is required for an extensive discharge clean in this order:

(1) Dispose of all disposable exposed equipment.
(2) Remove bed linen and fabric curtains.
(3) Thoroughly clean the bed, mattress, locker, cupboards and all horizontal surfaces at both high and low level.
(4) Clean the floor.
(5) Allow it to dry thoroughly.
(6) Remake the bed and restock the room.

Patient transfers
Patients in isolation should not leave the single/isolation room unless clinically essential. Portering staff should be advised of the infection control precautions needed. Protective clothing is only generally required when having direct contact with the patient. Isolated patients should not wait in communal patient waiting areas but should be transferred directly to the room in which a clinical intervention is taking place and be brought back to the isolation/single room directly. Trolleys or chairs used to transport patients should be decontaminated before further use.

THE PSYCHOLOGICAL CARE OF ISOLATED PATIENTS
Placing patients in single or isolation rooms segregates them from other patients, staff and the normal day-to-day activities on a ward. This forced segregation can be detrimental to the patient's psychological condition (Davies and Rees, 2000). Patients in isolation can experience a range of undesirable emotions (see Box 14.1 below).

After a decision has been made to isolate a patient, this should be discussed with the patient and relatives, where appropriate, as soon as possible. Written information leaflets are useful to

---

**Box 14.1   Emotions patients can experience
when isolated (Ward, 2000).**

- Frustration
- Loneliness
- Neglect
- Stigmatisation
- Abandonment
- Depression
- Anxiety
- Boredom
- Confinement

---

explain the process of isolation, as both patients and relatives can forget verbal information given at a stressful time.

The environment of isolation is important to the patient's experience. Patients and relatives class the following as important in improving the experience of isolation:

- Regular contact with the staff
- Good communication and up-to-date information
- A good level of cleanliness in the room
- Flexible visiting times
- Access to newspapers, television and/or radio
- Access to a telephone
- Activities to pass the time. (Rees *et al.*, 2000; Ward, 2000)

Staff caring for isolated patients need to ensure they have the skills and abilities to provide optimum care to these patients whilst they are in a vulnerable situation. In particular, nursing staff should consider the following when caring for isolated patients:

- Appropriate information must be given to both the patient and relatives before isolation wherever possible and updated on a regular basis.
- Isolated patients should have access to call bells to alert staff promptly when they require assistance.
- Nursing staff should endeavour to enter the isolation room regularly, even if the patient requires no specific care at that time.

- Single/isolation room furniture should be arranged to enable patients to see out of doors and windows easily.
- Visiting should be encouraged but nursing staff should also ensure that the patient is not becoming too tired or exhausted due to an excessive numbers of visitors.
- The patient's psychological well-being should be assessed on a regular basis.
- Nurses caring for isolated patients should ensure that they are competent in identifying mood disturbances and discriminating between depression and anxiety.
- Where existing clinical staff are unable to provide the appropriate psychological care for patients suffering psychological effects such as depression or anxiety, assistance should be sought from appropriately qualified personnel, for example psychologists.
- Nursing staff should ensure that housekeeping activities, such as cleaning, meal and drink provision and meal tray clearance occur.
- Patients should be provided with access to telephones, televisions and reading material as required.
- Nursing staff should ensure that patients receive rehabilitation activities where this is essential to the patient's continued recovery and well-being. (Gammon, 1999; Rees *et al.*, 2000; Ward, 2000)

SCENARIO

A 65-year-old man who has undergone a cardiac bypass graft is found to have MRSA in his sternal wound. What are the isolation requirements in terms of preventing spread of infection and what are the important aspects of isolation care that will now be required?

Isolation in a single room with en suite facilities, if possible, is required. The door should be kept shut where possible and must be closed during bedmaking and wound dressing procedures. Staff will wear gloves and aprons on entering the room. The patient and relatives should be advised of why single room isolation is needed and given written information regarding this. Nursing staff should ensure that the patient has a call bell and access to recreational activities such as television, books and newspapers.

SUMMARY

Isolation of patients to prevent spread of infection should be preceded by a risk assessment that includes not only infection risk but also clinical risk to the patient. Once a decision has been made to isolate, patients are generally placed in either a single room or a specifically designed isolation room and good principles for isolation are followed. Care and management should address the information and psychological needs of the patient and their relatives. Providing practical support, including access to televisions and telephones can help to reduce the psychological effects of isolation.

REFERENCES

Davies, H. and Rees, J. (2000) Psychological effects of isolation nursing (1) mood disturbance. *Nursing Standard*, **14** (28), 35–38.

Gammon, J. (1999) Isolated instance. *Nursing Times*, **95** (2), 57–60.

Garner, J.S. and the Hospital Infection Control Practices Advisory Committee (1996) Guideline for isolation precautions in hospitals. *American Journal of Infection Control*, **24**, 24–52.

Gopal Rao, G. and Jeanes, A. (1999) A pragmatic approach to the use of isolation facilities. *Bugs and Drugs*, **5** (1), 4–6.

NHS Estates (2002) *Infection Control in the Built Environment*. The Stationery Office, London.

NHS Estates (2004) *Total Waste Management: Best Practice Advice on Local Waste Management for the NHS in England*. Available from: http://195.92.246.148/knowledge_network/documents/Waste_strategy_20041028144518.pdf (accessed 20 November 2006).

NHS Executive (1995) *Hospital Laundry Arrangements for Used and Infected Linen* (HSG(95)18). NHS Executive, London.

Rees, J., Davies, H., Birchall, C. and Price, J. (2000) Psychological effects of source isolation nursing (2) patient satisfaction. *Nursing Standard*, **14** (29), 32–36.

Ward, D. (2000) Infection control: reducing the psychological effects of isolation. *British Journal of Nursing*, **9** (3), 162–170.

The Immunocompromised Patient

15

INTRODUCTION

Patients may be immunocompromised due to innate inadequacies in their immune system, the effects of specific diseases and the effects of treatments used for certain conditions and diseases. Patients with compromised immune systems are at increased risk from infections that can affect any patient in hospital, but they are also at risk from infections that do not generally affect patients with adequate immunity. In the absence of an adequate immune response to infection, it is even more important that infection prevention measures are strictly applied. This chapter details the infection prevention requirements of patients who are severely immunocompromised.

LEARNING OBJECTIVES
By the end of this chapter you will be able to:

❏ Describe what is meant by opportunistic infections and the types of infections that can affect immunocompromised patients
❏ Discuss the additional infection prevention precautions required for this patient group

CONDITIONS THAT AFFECT THE IMMUNE SYSTEM
An adequately functioning immune system is necessary to protect us from the constant challenge that human beings are met with when in contact with micro-organisms. The immune system and the immune response to infection are covered in detail in Chapter 2. The key components of the immune system are:

- The non-specific immune functions, including the action of secretions, the inflammatory response and phagocytosis
- The specific immune functions, including the action of lymphocytes and killer cells

If any, or all, of these functions are not operating adequately then some degree of immunocompromise will be present. Severe immune deficiency can be innate (inborn) or can be acquired, either through disease processes or treatment effects.

Innate immune deficiency   is relatively rare. An example of this would be severe immune deficiency syndrome (SIDS), where a baby does not develop any immune function after birth.

Acquired immune deficiency through disease   can be specific to particular cells, for example human immunodeficiency virus, which affects numbers of T-lymphocytes.

Acquired immune deficiency through interventions   occurs when medications are given that affect the normal functioning of the immune system. Examples of this are chemotherapy treatments for cancer and anti-rejection therapy for transplant recipients.

CHANGING PATTERNS OF INFECTION

Patients with immune deficiency are at increased risk of infection from micro-organisms that are generally associated with hospital acquired infection. Gram positive micro-organisms, including *Staphylococcus aureus*, coagulase negative staphylococci and streptococci are commonly found to be causes of infection in oncology patients; Gram negative micro-organisms, including *Escherichia coli* can also be found causing infections in these patients (Urrea *et al.*, 2004). Outbreaks of methicillin resistant *Staphylococcus aureus* (MRSA) and *Clostridium difficile* have been reported in oncology and bone marrow transplant units (Moore, 2005; Gross *et al.*, 2006). In addition to these common hospital infections, opportunistic infections (those that do not normally cause infection in individuals with adequate immune system) are found in immune deficient patients. These include fungal infections such as *Aspergillus* spp. (Lai, 2001), listeria (Barnett, 2000) and *Candida* spp. (Risi and Tomascak, 1998). Viral infections can also be problematic in units caring for immune deficient patients, for example adenovirus (Carriker *et al.*, 2005) and due to the lack of immune function these patients can excrete viruses for a considerably longer time than immunocompetent individuals. The administration of medications to suppress the immune response can also lead to the reactivation of dormant infections, for example cytomegalovirus.

PREVENTION OF INFECTION

The following principles for infection prevention apply to patients who have a severe risk of infection due to immune deficiency, for example those patients who have granulocyte levels of less than $0.5 \times 10^9/l$ (Wilson, 1995).

The environment

Patient placement will depend on the degree of a patient's immunodeficiency and the location in which the patient is to be cared for. For example, a patient with neutropenia on a general ward where MRSA is endemic should be placed in a single room to protect them from risk of infection. Patients who are undergoing bone marrow transplantation using cells from a donor will normally be cared for in protective isolation rooms with air filtration at the point of entry and positive air pressure within the room (Dykewicz and Kaplan, 2000). This level of protective isolation may not be necessary for other neutropenic patients, provided infection prevention and control procedures are adequate (Mank and van der Lelie, 2003). Patient placement is particularly important during construction and renovation activities as dust created during these activities has the potential to lead to invasive *Aspergillus* spp. infection (NHS Estates, 2002).

A high standard of environmental cleanliness is essential. Wards and units caring for immune deficient patients should be classified as very high risk for cleaning and monitoring purposes (see Chapter 16 for detailed guidance on cleaning risk classification and cleaning specifications). No unnecessary items which could contribute to dust collection should be kept in patient rooms. Flowers and pot plants should not be permitted in wards or units for immune deficient patients (Risi and Tomascak, 1998). Carpets should not be installed adjacent to protective isolation rooms, as these have been associated with aspergillosis (Gerson *et al.*, 1994).

Hand hygiene

Adherence to good hand hygiene is essential (Risi and Tomascak, 1998). Antimicrobial soaps are recommended if hands are being washed (Dykewicz and Kaplan, 2000); alcohol hand rubs are acceptable provided hands are not visibly contaminated with organic matter (Pratt *et al.*, 2007). All persons entering the room of an immune deficient patient, both staff and relatives, should decontaminate their hands before entering and on leaving.

Protective clothing

Staff entering protective isolation rooms should wear gloves and aprons in accordance with standard precaution guidelines. Storage or protective clothing should be in a clean area as inappropriate storage can lead to contamination of plastic aprons (Callaghan, 1998). Guidance on choice of sterile or non-sterile gloves is given in Chapter 5. However, gloves in dispenser boxes have been found to be contaminated with both spore and non-spore forming bacteria including *Bacillus cereus* (Berthelot *et al.*, 2006). As immune deficient patients are more susceptible to opportunistic infection activities in which non-sterile gloves are used for immunocompetent patients they might require the use of sterile gloves in, for example, invasive device handling.

Food and water

Water and ice have been associated with outbreaks of infection in immune deficient patients (Stout *et al.*, 1985; Communicable Disease Review, 1993). Drinks and ice made from tap water should be avoided by patients with severe immune deficiency; boiled, cooled water can be used for cold drinks. Ice-making machines in wards and units for immune deficient patients should be on a regular cleaning schedule (Barnett, 2000). The following food products have been associated with infections that may be particularly hazardous in the immune deficient patient:

- Uncooked vegetables and salads – *Escherichia coli*, *Salmonella* spp., *Listeria* spp.
- Soft and blue cheeses – *Listeria* spp., fungi
- Unpasteurised dairy products – *Campylobacter*, *Listeria* spp.
- Eggs – *Salmonella* spp. (Manojlovic, 2003)

Severely immune deficient patients should avoid these foods, particularly when they are raw. Good food hygiene, including hand hygiene, appropriate segregation and storage of food, and adequate cooking of food is essential when meeting the dietary needs of immune deficient patients. Food prepared outside the hospital should not be given to neutropenic patients (Risi and Tomascak, 1998) to reduce the risk of gastroenteritis.

Visitors

Visitors should be advised of the infection control procedures in place, particularly hand hygiene. A process should be in place to ask visitors whether they have had contact with any infections before they visit. In particular, checks should be made for the following, and exclusion from visiting considered, for bone marrow transplant patients:

- Upper respiratory tract infections
- Flu-like illness
- Chickenpox
- Shingles
- Oral polio vaccination in the preceding 3–6 weeks
- Diarrhoea and/or vomiting
- German measles
- Unexplained rash and fever
- Whooping cough
- Group A streptococcal pharyngitis (Dykewicz and Kaplan, 2000; Risi and Tomascak, 1998)

Children should be able to comply with the infection prevention procedure required, for example adequate hand hygiene. Careful screening of children's infectious status and their contact with potentially infectious diseases should take place even if they appear to be healthy (Risi and Tomascak, 1998).

Staff

Staff caring for immune deficient patients should be up to date with their vaccinations. Staff with diseases that are transmitted by air, droplet and direct contact should not have direct contact with immune deficient patients. In particular, staff should be excluded if they have:

- Infectious gastroenteritis
- Flu-like illness
- Upper respiratory infections
- Shingles
- Herpes simplex virus lesions on lips or hands (Dykewicz and Kaplan, 2000)

Selective decontamination of the gut

The gut may be an important source of infection in neutropenic patients where no obvious source of infection can be identified (Schimpff *et al.*, 1972). The administration of antibiotics that do not affect the normal gut bacteria has been used for neutropenic patients but the widespread use of this is questionable due to the risk of bacterial resistance developing (Risi and Tomascak, 1998).

SCENARIO

When caring for a 35-year-old lady who is in protective isolation having undergone a donor bone marrow transplant, what are the key factors that nursing staff should consider when entering her isolation room?

Nursing staff should not enter the room if they have an infectious disease that could be readily transmitted to the patient. Hands should be decontaminated and the appropriate protective clothing worn. Any reusable equipment that is to be taken into the room should be checked to ensure that it has been adequately decontaminated.

SUMMARY

Patients with compromised immune systems may be susceptible to infections from micro-organisms that are not pathogenic in other individuals. Additional infection prevention activities may be needed to protect them from infections from visitors, staff and the environment. Strict adherence to infection prevention activities is vital in units caring for immunocompromised patients.

REFERENCES

Barnett, J. (2000) Immunosuppressed patients. In: *Infection Control; Science, Management and Practice* (ed. J. McCulloch). Whurr Publishers, London.

Berthelot, P., Dietmann, J., Fascia, P. *et al.* (2006) *American Journal of Infection Control*, **34**, 128–130.

Callaghan, I. (1998) Bacterial contamination of nurses' uniforms: a study. *Nursing Standard*, **13** (1), 37–42.

Carriker, C., McDonald, J., Oden, M., Engemann, J. and Kaye, K. (2005) Striking a balance between freedom and safety on a pediatric bone marrow transplant unit. *American Journal of Infection Control*, **33** (35), 95.

Communicable Disease Review (1993) Ice as a source of infection acquired in hospital. *Communicable Disease Review Weekly*, **3** (53), 241.

Dykewicz, C.A., Kaplan, J.E. and the Guidelines Working Group Members from the CDC, the Infectious Disease Society of America, and the American Society of Blood and Marrow Transplantation (2000) *Morbidity and Mortality Weekly Review*, **49**, 1–128.

Gerson, S.L., Parker, P., Jacobs, M.R., Creger, R. and Lazarus, H.M. (1994) Aspergillosis due to carpet contamination. *Infection Control Hospital Epidemiology*, **15**, 221–223.

Gross, M.A., Fauerbach, L.L., Ruse, M.T., Kelly, R.E. and Archibald, L.K. (2006) *Clostridium difficile* disease in bone marrow transplant unit. *American Journal of Infection Control*, June, 141.

Lai, K.K. (2001) A cluster of invasive aspergillosis in a bone marrow transplant unit related to construction and the utility of air sampling. *American Journal of Infection Control*, **29**, 333–337.

Mank, A. and van der Lelie, H. (2003) Is there still an indication for nursing patients with prolonged neutropenia in protective isolation? An evidence based nursing and medical study of four years' experience for nursing patients with neutropenia without isolation. *European Journal of Oncology Nursing*, **7** (1), 17–23.

Manojlovic, G. (2003) Immunosuppressive diseases. In: *Infection Control in the Community* (eds J. Lawrence and D. May). Churchill Livingstone, Edinburgh.

Moore, L. (2005) Cluster of methicillin resistant *Staphylococcus aureus* (MRSA) on an oncology unit: identification, investigation and correction. *American Journal of Infection Control*, **33** (35), 96.

NHS Estates (2002) *Infection Control in the Built Environment*. The Stationery Office, London.

Pratt, R.J., Pellowe, C.M., Wilson, J.A., Loveday, H.P., Jones, S.R., McDougall, C. and Wilcox, M.H. (2007) epic2: national evidence based guidelines for preventing healthcare associated infections in NHS hospitals in England. *Journal of Hospital Infection*, **65** (Suppl. 1, Feb.), S1–64.

Risi, G.F. and Tomascak, V. (1998) Prevention of infection in the immunocompromised host. *American Journal of Infection Control*, **26**, 594–606.

Schimpff, S.C., Young, V.M., Vermeulen, G.D., Moody. M.R. and Wiernik, P.H. (1972) Origin of infection in acute non-lymphocytic leukaemia: significance of hospital acquisition of potential pathogens. *Annals of Internal Medicine*, **77**, 707–714.

Stout, J.E., Victor, L.Y. and Mucara, P. (1985) Isolation of *Legionella pneumophila* from the cold water of hospital ice machines: implications for the origin and transmission of the organism. *Infection Control*, **6** (4), 141–146.

Urrea, M., Rives, S., Cruz, O., Navarro, A., Garcia, J.J. and Estella, J. (2004) *American Journal of Infection Control*, **32**, 205–208.

Wilson, J. (1995) *Infection Control in Clinical Practice.* Baillière Tindall, London.

Decontamination

16

INTRODUCTION

Equipment that is used for more than one patient needs adequate decontamination between each use to prevent spread of infection. The environment in which care is provided should be of a standard of cleanliness acceptable to patients. This chapter covers principles of decontamination, risk assessment and processes used for decontamination of equipment and the environment.

LEARNING OBJECTIVES

By the end of this chapter you will be able to:

❑ Define decontamination, cleaning, sterilisation and disinfection
❑ Describe common processes that are used for decontamination of equipment and the environment
❑ State appropriate decontamination processes for some commonly used healthcare equipment
❑ Understand the nursing contribution to a clean healthcare environment

DECONTAMINATION PROCESSES

Decontamination is the term used to describe a variety of methods that can be used to render a piece of medical equipment safe for use. Decontamination can be achieved by using one or more of the following processes:

• Cleaning
• Disinfection
• Sterilisation

Cleaning is a physical process that removes soil and organic matter and some micro-organisms from a device. Cleaning is a prerequisite to disinfection and sterilisation. Cleaning can be undertaken either by hand or by machine. Cleaning by hand can be defined further into immersion (where the device is cleaned underwater) or non-immersion. Hand washing of items should only be undertaken if it is not possible to use an automated process. With any manual cleaning process there are risks associated with the cleaning chemical being used as well as with micro-organisms that could be present on the device being cleaned. Protective clothing in the form of gloves, apron or gown and eye protection (where appropriate) should be worn.

Process for manual cleaning – immersion

- Don appropriate protective clothing.
- Fill sink with sufficient warm water and detergent solution (at the appropriate dilution) to cover the item to be washed.
- Immerse the item in water, ensuring that the solution reaches all appropriate parts.
- Brush, wipe or agitate the item to remove all visible soiling, ensuring the item remains under water.
- Transfer the item to a clean sink or receptacle and rinse with clean water.
- Remove item from rinse water and drain.
- Dry item thoroughly with non-shedding absorbent cloth.

Process for manual cleaning – non-immersion

- If the item is electrical, ensure it is not connected to the mains supply.
- Don appropriate protective clothing.
- Fill sink with sufficient warm water and detergent solution at the appropriate dilution.
- Immerse a clean, disposable, non-shedding cloth in the detergent solution and wring thoroughly.
- Starting with the upper surface, wipe thoroughly ensuring that water does not enter electrical components.
- Periodically rinse the cloth in clean water, re-immerse in the detergent solution and wring thoroughly.

- Dry item thoroughly with non-shedding absorbent cloth.
- An alcohol wipe may be used to assist the drying process.

Mechanical cleaning can be undertaken in a washer-disinfector, with a heat disinfection programme, or an ultrasonic washer. Ultrasonic washers use an agitation process to remove dirt and soil. Automated washing equipment should only be operated by staff trained in its use and it must undergo regular testing and maintenance.

Disinfection reduces the number of infectious agents present on an item but does not necessarily inactivate certain microorganisms, including some viruses and bacterial spores. Disinfection can be achieved by the use of chemicals or by heat. A heat process is preferred as there is more control in the process and exposure of staff to hazardous chemicals is reduced. Heat disinfection can be achieved by the use of a thermal washer-disinfector or by low temperature steam. The lower the temperature in one of these processes, the longer it will take to achieve disinfection. If a temperature of 73°C is achieved, disinfection will be achieved in three minutes. If a temperature of 60°C is achieved, it will take ten minutes to achieve disinfection. Machinery used for thermal or low temperature steam disinfection should only be operated by trained staff and it must undergo regular testing and maintenance.

Chemical disinfection is less reliable than heat disinfection as it depends on the right concentration of disinfectant being used, as well as on the item being in contact with the disinfectant for an appropriate time. It should only be used where an item of equipment cannot tolerate disinfection by heat. Chemical disinfectants have varying spectrums of activity against microorganisms. Table 16.1 shows this varying activity.

When using chemical disinfectants it is important to pay attention to safety aspects as some of these chemicals can be hazardous to staff. They should only be used with appropriate precautionary measures as determined by risk assessment in line with Control of Substances Hazardous to Health Regulations (Health and Safety Executive, 1999). Some chemical disinfectants can cause damage to certain components in medical devices. Compatibility of the

Table 16.1 Microbial activity of disinfectants (adapted from Medical Devices Agency, 2002a).

Disinfectant	Bacteria	Mycobacteria	Spores	Viruses
Alcohol	Good	Moderate	None	Moderate
Gluteraldehyde	Good	Good	Poor	Good
Chlorine dioxide	Good	Good	Good	Good
Peracetic acid	Good	Good	Good	Good
Superoxidised saline	Good	Good	Good	Good
Orthophthaldehyde	Good	Good	Poor	Good

disinfectant with the item being processed should be checked (Medical Devices Agency, 2001).

Sterilisation is the complete removal of all infectious agents from an item, including viruses and bacterial spores. Sterilisation can be achieved by dry heat, steam under pressure, gas or radiation. Dry heat requires temperatures in excess of 160°C and so is not suitable for items that will be damaged by these extreme temperatures. Sterilisation by steam under pressure is commonly used for medical devices, including surgical instruments. Autoclaving is a term often used for this method of decontamination. Items must be able to withstand temperatures in the region of 134°C. Small bench-top autoclave sterilisers are sometimes used in community settings, including general practices and dental surgeries. If they do not have a vacuum cycle to remove air, they are not suitable for sterilisation of items that have lumens or channels as the steam will not penetrate into these small channels. Large autoclave sterilisers are generally found in sterile supplies departments within hospitals. They are suitable for processing most items that can withstand high temperatures.

Gas plasma is an emerging technology that can be used to sterilise items that are not heat tolerant. Ethylene oxide sterilisation is a technique that has been in use for some time. It is a hazardous process that is only available in a limited number of locations in the UK. Items sterilised by this method have to be contained in a holding area after processing until residual gas has been released from sterilised items. Sterilisation by irradiation is generally used for pre-packaged, single use items that are commercially prepared, for example syringes and needles.

DETERMINING WHICH PROCESS TO USE
The decontamination process for individual items is determined by the intended use. Medical devices can be classified according to the infection risk associated with their use (Babb, 2000).

High risk items   are those that are used in a sterile body area or are in contact with a break in the skin or mucous membranes. An example of equipment in this risk category is surgical instruments. Sterilisation is required. In exceptional circumstances, for example flexible endoscopes used in procedures such as gastroscopy, disinfection may be acceptable.

Intermediate risk items   are those that have contact with intact mucous membranes, body fluids, or are contaminated with highly transmissible micro-organisms. An example of an item in this category is a laryngoscope blade. Items to be used non-invasively on patients at increased risk of infection may fall into this category. Disinfection is required for these items.

Low risk items   are in contact with intact skin. An example of an item in this category is a blood pressure monitoring cuff. Cleaning is usually adequate for these items, but disinfection may be needed if there is the risk that they have been contaminated with specific micro-organisms, for example *Clostridium difficile*.

Minimal risk items   are not in close contact with patients or their immediate surroundings. These items would include trolley surfaces and floors. It is usually adequate to clean items in this category.
    The following algorithm is helpful in determining the appropriate decontamination method (see Figure 16.1).

ENVIRONMENTAL CLEANLINESS
Patients expect to be cared for in a clean safe environment. Nurses have a responsibility to ensure a ward or department is clean,

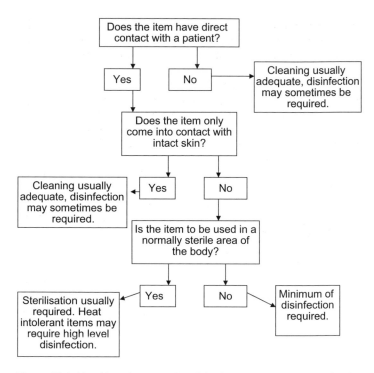

Figure 16.1 Algorithm for assessing infection risk and decontamination process.

even if they are not the person who is doing the actual cleaning (Jeanes, 2004). Items of equipment that come into direct contact with a patient are more likely to be responsible for transmission of infection; however, environmental contamination can be a source of infection (Rampling *et al.*, 2001).

DECONTAMINATION OF THE ENVIRONMENT
Although general cleaning tasks are often the responsibility of domestic and housekeeping staff, nursing staff need basic knowledge of cleaning procedures to enable them to monitor cleanli-

ness standards and where cleaning tasks are necessary in the absence of domestic staff. The following key principles should be applied to cleaning tasks in the clinical environment:

- Cleaning equipment should be clean and dry before use.
- Wear protective clothing as appropriate (e.g. gloves, aprons, eye protection) to protect against contact with hazardous chemicals.
- Always ventilate areas where chemicals are used.
- Clean from the highest to the lowest point and from the dirtiest to the cleanest point.
- Every effort should be made to create minimal dust during cleaning.
- Cleaning activities should not be carried out when invasive procedures and aseptic techniques are being performed in the immediate vicinity.
- Cleaning equipment is colour coded and should only be used for the areas allocated to the colour code as follows:

  — Red (disposable) – bathrooms, washrooms, showers, toilets, basins and bathroom floors
  — Blue – general areas including wards, departments, offices
  — Green – catering departments, ward kitchen areas and patient food services
  — Yellow – isolated areas (NPSA, 2007) surfaces
  — White (disposable) – isolation rooms, operating rooms and ante-rooms

- Mop heads should be removed and sent for laundering after use.
- All cleaning equipment should be adequately decontaminated, dried and stored in a manner to prevent contamination after each use; disposable equipment should be discarded. (NHS Estates, 2003)

DECONTAMINATION OF COMMONLY USED CLINICAL EQUIPMENT

Manufacturers' instructions for decontamination of medical devices and equipment should always be followed. Where a specific product or process is recommended, it should always be confirmed that this is available in the healthcare facility before equipment is purchased or used. When using chemicals it is important to check that the chemical is compatible with the medical device, as incompatibility can lead to problems such as corrosion (Medical Devices Agency, 2001). Table 16.2 gives guidance on decontamination processes for some commonly used medical and nursing equipment.

DECONTAMINATION OF ENDOSCOPES

Endoscopes are either rigid instruments with optical lenses or are flexible with fibre optics used for imaging. Rigid endoscopes are generally heat tolerant and should be sterilised by autoclaving. Flexible endoscopes are generally not heat tolerant and therefore cannot be sterilised by heat. Flexible scopes are used for many different purposes and the risk of infection will vary depending on the intended use of the scope. Infections with Gram negative bacteria, for example *Pseudomonas aeruginosa* can occur. Other infections that have been related to endoscopy include *Mycobacterium tuberculosis* (TB) and hepatitis B. Risk of Creutzfeldt-Jakob disease should also be considered during endoscopy as some procedures may involve contact with lymphoid tissue. High level disinfection is required for flexible scopes, that is the use of a disinfectant that can kill spores under certain circumstances, for example peracetic acid or chlorine dioxide.

Decontamination of endoscopes should only be undertaken by staff who have been appropriately trained and assessed as competent. The following general principles apply to decontamination and infection prevention for flexible endoscopes:

- Accessories used with flexible endoscopes should be heat tolerant and be sterilised by autoclaving.
- Flexible endoscopes should be processed immediately before intended use.
- Endoscopes must be cleaned before disinfection; an automated washing process should be used in preference to manual washing.
- Where automated washing and/or disinfection machines are used, it is important to ensure that the correct connectors are used and that all channels in the endoscopes are adequately disinfected.

Table 16.2 Decontamination of commonly used clinical equipment.

Equipment	Decontamination process
Bedframes	Clean with detergent and water between each patient use and at regular intervals for long-stay patients. Disinfection may be needed in certain circumstances, for example after an MRSA positive patient.
Bedpans and urinals	Reusable pans should be disinfected by heat between uses. Holders for disposable bedpans must at a minimum be cleaned between patient use.
Blood pressure cuff	Wipe between patient uses with detergent wipe. Some cuffs may be launderable.
Commodes	Clean with detergent and water between each patient use. Disinfection needed if contaminated with body fluid and in certain circumstances, for example after *Clostridium difficile* positive patient.
Dressing trolleys	Clean with detergent and water before each use.
Drip stand	Clean with detergent and water between each patient use and at regular intervals for long-stay patients. Disinfection may be needed in certain circumstances, for example after an MRSA positive patient.
Hoist sling	Dedicated to individual patient use. Reusable slings should be laundered at a minimum of 60°C between patient uses. Disposable slings may be used.
Infusion pump	Clean between patient use with detergent or alcohol wipe. Prolonged use of alcohol may cause hardening and cracking of plastic.
Mattress	Clean with detergent and water between each patient use and at regular intervals for long-stay patients. If disinfection is needed care must be taken to ensure the disinfectant does not affect the mattress cover properties. Specialist mattresses should undergo a decontamination process by the manufacturer or in a dedicated on-site facility.
Monitoring equipment	Clean between patient use with detergent or alcohol wipe. Prolonged use of alcohol may cause hardening and cracking of plastic.
Nebulisers	Individual patient use. During use cleaning may be needed. Sterile water should be used for cleaning to prevent risk of Legionnaire's disease.

Table 16.2 *Continued*

Equipment	Decontamination process
Patient tables and lockers	Clean with detergent and water between each patient use and at regular intervals for long-stay patients. Disinfection may be needed in certain circumstances, for example after an MRSA positive patient.
Patient wash bowls	Dedicate individual patient wash bowls wherever possible. Clean with detergent and water between each patient use. Disinfection may be needed in certain circumstances, for example after an MRSA positive patient.
Pillows	Clean with detergent and water between each patient use and at regular intervals for long-stay patients. Disinfection may be needed in certain circumstances, for example after an MRSA positive patient. Pillows should be fully enclosed in a waterproof cover.
Scissors	Clean with detergent and water. Sterile scissors should be used for aseptic procedures.
Sliding sheet	Dedicated to individual patient use. Reusable sheets should be laundered at a minimum of 60°C between patient uses. Disposable sheets may be used.
Stethoscope	Minimum of clean between each patient use.
Wheelchairs	Clean with detergent and water between each patient use and at regular intervals for long-stay patients. Disinfection may be needed in certain circumstances, for example after an MRSA positive patient.

- Endoscopes should be loaded into an automatic washer/disinfector to ensure that the disinfectant comes in contact with all external parts of the scope.
- Water used for rinsing after disinfection must be free of bacteria.
- After use, flexible scopes should be disinfected and stored in a vertical position in a ventilated cupboard. There is a risk of micro-organism growth in the channels during storage. Scopes

that have been stored for more than three hours should be disinfected again before use on a patient.

- Information should be recorded and stored as to which flexible endoscope and accessories are used on each patient in case there is a need to trace the use of a scope back to individual patients. (Medical Devices Agency, 2002b; Medicines and Healthcare Products Regulatory Agency, 2005; 2006a)

SINGLE USE EQUIPMENT

A single use item is generally intended for use on an individual patient for one procedure only and then discarded, for example indwelling urinary catheter. Single patient use items are generally intended for use on an individual patient only, but may be used more than once on the same patient, for example a nebuliser. Single use items are generally identified by labelling on packaging that states this or by the following symbol ②. Reprocessing a single use device against the directions of the manufacturer could lead to mechanical failure of the device as well as to transmission of infection if the device is inadequately decontaminated (Medicines and Healthcare Products Regulatory Agency, 2006h). It is also possible that legal liability, should the device fail in use, would pass to the healthcare organisation rather than the manufacturer. Healthcare staff should not reprocess single use items against the advice of their employers

DECONTAMINATION OF DEVICES
BEFORE INSPECTION AND REPAIR

Equipment that is being sent for service, maintenance or repair must be adequately decontaminated to prevent risk of infection to technical staff who may handle it. Before sending any medical equipment away from a ward or department, or allowing technical staff to handle medical equipment in a ward the item should be emptied of body fluids and adequately decontaminated using an appropriate process. It may be necessary to complete a certificate that details how the device has been decontaminated (DoH, 1993). Technical staff may refuse to handle equipment without this assurance. Occasionally, it may not be possible to fully decontaminate an item, for example if the item is damaged or if it is to be the subject of an investigation. In these circumstances it will be necessary to provide details of the likely sources and type of contamination that may be present on a piece of equipment.

SCENARIO

You are discharging a patient who has been on the ward for a period of one week. What are the decontamination requirements of the bed space before you can admit another patient?

First, all clinical waste and laundry should be discarded in line with hospital policy. All parts of the mattress, pillows and bed, including head and foot boards, bed rails etc., should be cleaned and dried. The locker should be checked for the presence of any patient items and then cleaned and dried, inside and out. The bed table should be cleaned. All other components in the bed space, including suction equipment, patient entertainment systems and documentation folders should also be cleaned. Curtains should be checked for signs of visible contamination and changed if there is visible soiling. If the patient has been subject to specific infection control precautions then disinfection may be needed and curtains may need to be changed.

SUMMARY

Adequate decontamination of medical equipment is important in prevention of infection. Decontamination is achieved by one or more processes including cleaning, disinfection and sterilisation. The intended use of an item determines the decontamination process that is needed.

REFERENCES

Babb, J. (2000) Decontamination of the environment, equipment and the skin. In: *Control of Hospital Infection: a Practical Handbook* (eds G.A.J. Ayliffe, A.P. Fraise, A.M. Geddes, and K. Mitchell). Arnold, London.

Department of Health (1993) *HSG(93)26 Decontamination of Equipment Prior to Inspection, Service or Repair.* Department of Health, London.

Health and Safety Executive (1999) *Control of Substances Hazardous to Health (COSHH) (Amendments) Act.* Health and Safety Executive, London.

Jeanes, A. (2004) Keeping hospitals clean: how nurses can reduce healthcare associated infection. *Professional Nurse,* **20** (6), 35.

Medical Devices Agency (2001) *SN 2001(28) Compatibility of Medical Devices and Reprocessing Equipment with Decontaminating Agents.* Medical Devices Agency, London.

Medical Devices Agency (2002a) *Microbiological Advisory Committee Manual – Part 1 – Principles.* Medical Devices Agency, London.

Medical Devices Agency (2002b) *DB 2002(05) Decontamination of Endoscopes.* Medical Devices Agency, London.

Medicine and Healthcare Products Regulatory Agency (2005) *Top Ten Tips: Endoscope Decontamination.* Medicine and Healthcare Products Regulatory Agency, London.

Medicine and Healthcare Products Regulatory Agency (2006a) *Microbiological Advisory Committee Manual – Part 3 – Procedures.* Medicine and Healthcare Products Regulatory Agency, London.

Medicine and Healthcare Products Regulatory Agency (2006b) *DB 2006(04) Single Use Medical Devices: Implications and Consequences of Reuse.* Medicine and Healthcare Products Regulatory Agency, London.

National Patient Safety Agency (2007) *Safer practice notice 15: colour coding hospital cleaning materials and equipment.* National Patient Safety Agency, London.

NHS Estates (2003) *Healthcare Facilities Cleaning Manual* Available at: http://patientexperience.nhsestates.gov.uk/clean_hospitals/ch_content/cleaning_manual/background.asp#introduction (accessed 23 November 2006).

Rampling, A., Wiseman, S., Davis, L. *et al.* (2001) Evidence that hospital hygiene is important in the control of methicillin resistant *Staphylococcus aureus. Journal of Hospital Infection*, **49** (2), 109–116.

Index

Page entries for headings with subheadings refer to general aspects of that topic
Page entries shown in **bold** denote boxes/figures/tables

Adenovirus, **217**
Administration set management, 172, **173**
Aids/HIV, 3, 66, 85, 110, 246
Airborne infections, 254, 257
Allergies, 77–78
Anaesthesia, 220–22, **223**, 231
Antibiotics, *see* Chemotherapy, antimicrobial
Antibodies/immunoglobulins, 34–35, **35**
Anxiety, isolated patients, **264**
Aprons, 78–79, *see also* Protective clothing
Aseptic technique, intravascular therapy, 157
Aspergillus, **22**, 269
Autoclaves, 278; *see also* Decontamination
Avian influenza, patient isolation requirements, **259**

Bacteria, 14–18, **14**, **18**; *see also* Chemotherapy; Micro-organisms
Binary fission, bacteria, **17**/17
Blood, 62
    cultures, specimen collection, 47–50
    infections, 163, 166, 246–48
    spills, 90–91
Breast milk, 201–3
Bronchiolitis, 203–7, **259**
Burns units, 244–46

Campylobacter gastroenteritis, 271, **259**
Candida spp., **22**, 68, 156, 269
Cannulation, 59
Cardiothoracic units, 242–44
Catheters
    central venous (CVCs), 166–69
    complications, 164, 166, 169, 170
    epidural, 59, 221–22
    insertion principles, 163–64, 165, 167, 169
    management, 164, 165, 167–68, 170
    midline, 163–64

    peripheral arterial, 164–66
    peripherally inserted central venous, 169–70
    removal, 164, 166, 168–169, 170
    routes of infection, 155–56
    urinary, *see* Urinary catheter care
Catheter associated urinary tract infection (CAUTI), 141
Cell-mediated immunity, 35–36
Cell structure, bacterial, 14–16, **14**
Central venous catheters, 166–69
Chemotherapy, antimicrobial, 25–26, 60, 160
    bacterial resistance, 26–29, **28**, **29**, 97, 111; *see also* MRSA
Chemotherapy patients, isolation, 254
Chest drains, 244
Chickenpox (*Varicella zoster*), 207–11, **259**, 271
Children in hospital, *see* Paediatric settings
CJD (Creutzfeldt-Jakob disease), *see* TSE
Cleaning, 275, 276–77; *see also* Decontamination
    chickenpox infections, 209
    CJD/TSE infections, 124, **125**
    Clostridium difficile infections, 108
    environmental, 90, 279–81
    equipment, 275, 276–77
    ESBL infections, 130–1
    glycopeptide resistant enterococci infections, 119
    measles infections, 215
    MRSA, 101, **102–3**
    mumps infections, 212
    norovirus infections, 134
    and patient isolation, 262–63
    respiratory syncytial virus infections, 206
    tuberculosis infections, 114
Clostridium difficile, **18**, 5, 105–10, 233–34, **259**, 268
Clothing, protective, *see* Protective clothing

Collection, specimens, 38–40
Conjugation, bacterial, 27, **28**
Contamination incidents, sharps, 84–86, **85**
Coxsackie virus, **217**
CR-BSI (blood stream infection), 163, 166
Creutzfeldt-Jakob disease (CJD), *see* TSE
CVCs (central venous catheters), 166–67

Deceased patients, handling procedures
chickenpox infections, 211
CJD/TSE infections, 126
Clostridium difficile infections, 110
ESBL infections, 132
glycopeptide resistant enterococci infections, 21
measles infections, 216
meningitis infections, 128
MRSA infections, 105
mumps infections, 214
respiratory syncytial virus infections, 207
tuberculosis infections, 116
Decontamination, 68–69, 158, 272; *see also* Hand hygiene; *and see below*
Decontamination, equipment, 275, 286; *see also* Cleaning; for specific situations *see* Equipment care
anaesthetic equipment, 222, **223**
clinical equipment, 281–82, **283–84**
deciding on appropriate process, 279, **280**
disinfection, 275, 277–78
disinfectant effectiveness/uses, **278**
endoscopes, 282, 284–85
environmental cleanliness, 279–80
environmental decontamination, 280–81
equipment repairs, 285–86
single use equipment, 285
sterilisation, 275, 278–79
Depression, isolated patients, **264**
Dialysis, 248–50
Diarrhoea, infective, *see Clostridium difficile*; Gastroenteritis
Discharge from hospital, patient procedures
chickenpox infections, 211
CJD/TSE infections, 126
Clostridium difficile infections, 109–10
ESBLS infections, 132
glycopeptide resistant enterococci infections, 120
measles infections, 216

MRSA infections, 104–5
mumps infections, 214
norovirus infections, 135–36
respiratory syncytial virus infections, 207
tuberculosis infections, 116
Disinfectant effectiveness/uses, **278**; *see also* Decontamination
Disinfection, 201, 275, 277–78; *see also* Decontamination
Dressings, 160, 190–93

ELISA (Enzyme-linked immunosorbent assay), 24–25
Endoscopes, decontamination, 282, 284–85
Enteral feeding, 177–81
Enterococcus spp., 116–21, **117**, 177–79, 221
Environment, 90, 198–99, 269–70, 279–81; *see also* Cleaning; Decontamination
Environmental Protection Act and Controlled Waste Regulations (DoE, 1991), 86
Enzyme-linked immunosorbent assay (ELISA), 24–25
Epidural catheters, 59, 221–22
Equipment care; *see also* Decontamination, equipment
chickenpox infections, 210
CJD/TSE infections, 125
Clostridium difficile infections, 108
enteral feeding, 179
ESBL infections, 131
glycopeptide resistant enterococci infections, 119
intensive care units, 241–42
intravascular therapy, 159, 173–174
isolated patients, 261–62
measles infections, 215
meningitis infections, 127
MRSA infections, 103
mumps infections, 212
norovirus infections, 134
respiratory syncytial virus infections, 206
TSE infections, **235**, 236
tuberculosis infections, 114
ESBLs (Extended spectrum beta-lactamase producing Gram negatives), 128–31, **259**
Escherechia coli, **18**
and immunocompromised patients, 268, 271
and intravascular therapy, 156
patient isolation requirements, **259**
and urinary catheterisation, 144

Index

Escherechia coli, (*cont'd*)
  and VAP, 240
  wounds, 188
Extended spectrum beta-lactamase
    producing Gram negatives,
    128–31, **259**
Eye protection, 81

Face-masks, 79–81, **81**, 130, 198; *see also*
    Protective clothing
Faecal specimens, 46–47
Fatal familial insomnia, *see* TSE
Feed, enteral, 179–81; *see also* Food;
    Formula feeds; Milk preparation;
    Nutritional care
Feeding tubes, 182; *see also* Nutritional
    care
Food, 3, 78, 270; *see also* Feed; Milk
    preparation; Nutritional care
Formula feeds, 201
Freezers, 202–3
Fungal infections, 21–22, **22**, 68, 269

Gas plasma technology, 278; *see also*
    Decontamination
Gastroenteritis, 233–34, **259**, 271; *see
    also* Norovirus
Genetic mutation, bacteria, 27
German measles (*Rubella*), **259**, 271
Gerstmann Straussler-Scheinker
    syndrome, *see* TSE
Gloves, protective, 74–78, **75**, **76**, 157;
    see also Protective clothing
Gloving procedures, 228–29
Glycopeptide resistant enterococci
    (GRE), 116–21, **117**
Gowns, 78–79, 227–28; *see also*
    Protective clothing
GRE (Glycopeptide resistant
    enterococci), 116–21, **117**

Hand foot and mouth disease, **217**
Hand hygiene, 67–69, **70**
  chickenpox infections, 209
  CJD/TSE infections, 123
  Clostridium difficile infections, 108
  compliance, 73–74
  ESBL infections, 130
  glycopeptide resistant enterococci
    infections, 118
  and hand care, 71–73
  and immunocompromised patients,
    270
  intravascular therapy, 157, 159
  isolated patient care, 258
  measles infections, 215
  meningitis infections, 127
  MRSA infections, 97, 101

mumps infections, 212, 214
norovirus infections, 134
patients, 73
resident organisms, 68, 71
respiratory syncytial virus infections,
    205–6, 207
surgical hand preparation, 226–27
techniques, 69–71, **72**
transient organisms, 68
tuberculosis infections, 114, 115
Hazardous Waste Regulations (2005),
    86
Health Act (DoH, 2006), 4
Health and Safety at Work Act (HSE,
    2003), 4
Hepatitis, 66
  infection process, 32
  patient isolation requirements, **259**
  protective clothing, 92
  renal care, 246
  sharps injuries, 85
Historical perspectives, 1–3
HIV/Aids, 3, 66, 85, 110, 246
Hospital acquired infections, 5–7, **7**
Humoral immunity, 34–35

Ice, infection risk from, 270
Immune response, 32–34; *see also*
    Micro-organisms
  antibodies/immunoglobulins, 34–35,
    35
  cell-mediated immunity, 35–36
  complement system, 34
  first line of defence, 32–33
  humoral immunity, 34–35
Immune system deficiency, innate/
    acquired, 60, 267–68; *see also*
    HIV/Aids
Immunisation, 36
Immunocompromised patients, 267–73
Immunodeficiency, 60, 267–68; *see also*
    HIV/Aids
Immunoglobulins, 34–35, **35**
Impetigo, **217**
Implanted venous access ports, 170–71
Infection control principles, 66–67, 86–
    87, 90–92; *see also* Hand hygiene;
    Linen handling; Protective
    clothing; Sharps; Waste handling
Infection control nurses, 8, 9–10
Infection control structures/roles, 7–10
Infection processes, 31–32
Infectious parotitis *see mumps*
Infective diarrhoea, *see Clostridium
    difficile*; Viral gastroenteritis
Inflammatory response, 33
Influenza, patient isolation
    requirements, **259**

Intensive care units, 239–42
Intravascular therapy, 154–58, 160, 174;
    see also Catheters; Peripheral
    venous cannulae
  administration set management, 172,
    173
  associated devices, 171–74, **173**
  changing fluid bags, 172
  complications, 162–64, 166, 169–71
  documentation, 160–61, 162
  drug/equipment preparation, 159,
    173–174
  implanted venous access ports,
    170–71
Intubation infection risks, 59
Isolation, patient, 1, 254–5, 266; see also
    Patient placement (for specific
    infections)
  airborne infections, 254, 257
  cleaning/hygiene, 258, 262–63
  facilities, **256**, 256–57
  patient isolation precaution signs,
    257, **260**
  negative/positive pressure rooms,
    256–57, **258**, **259**
  paediatric settings, 198
  patient care equipment, 261–62
  patient placement, 257, **259**
  patient transfers, 263
  protective clothing, 258, 261
  psychological care, 255, 263–65, **264**

Kuru, see TSE

Laboratory tests, micro-organisms, 23–
    25, **24**, **25**
Latex allergies, 77–78
Linen handling, 87–88
  chickenpox infections, 210
  CJD/TSE infections, 125
  Clostridium difficile infections, 109
  ESBL infections, 131
  glycopeptide resistant enterococci
    infections, 119
  isolated patients, 262
  local laundry facilities, 89
  measles infections, 215
  meningitis infections, 127
  MRSA infections, 103
  mumps infections, 213
  norovirus infections, 135
  principles for safe handling, 88–89
  respiratory syncytial virus infections,
    206
  tuberculosis infections, 114
  uniforms, 89–90
Listeria spp., 269, 271
Loneliness, isolated patients, 198, **264**

Masks, face, 79–81, **81**, 130, 198; see also
    Protective clothing
Measles, 214–16, **259**; see also German
    measles
Meningitis, meningococcal, 126–28,
    259
Meticillin resistant *Staphylococcus
    aureus see* MRSA
Micro-organisms, 13–14, 37; see also
    Bacteria; Chemotherapy; Immune
    response
  fungi, 21–22, **22**
  infection process, 31–32
  and intravascular therapy, 156
  laboratory detection methods, 23–25,
    24, **25**
  protozoa, 22–23
  transmission routes, 29–31
  viruses, 18–21, **19**, **21**
  wound infecting, 188
Microscopy, 23
Midline catheters, 163–64
Milk preparation, 200–3
MRSA (Meticillin resistant
    Staphylococcus aureus), 96–97
  cleaning procedures, 101, **102–3**
  deceased patients, 105
  decolonisation, 100
  dialysis, 248
  hand hygiene, 97, 101
  and immunocompromised patients,
    268
  and intravascular therapy, 156
  patient discharge, 104–5
  patient isolation requirements
  patient placement/isolation, 98–99,
    104, 257, **259**, 269
  and peri-operative care 231–32
  protective clothing, 101
  screening, for, 99–100
  specimen collection, 51–52
  treatment, 100–1
  and VAP, 240
  visitors, 104
  wounds, 188
Multi-drug resistant tuberculosis
    (MDR-TB), 110–11, **259**; see also
    Tuberculosis
Multi-resistant bacteria, 231–32, 254;
    see also ESBLs; MRSA; Multi-drug
    resistant tuberculosis
Mumps, 212–14, **259**
Myobacterium tuberculosis, see
    Tuberculosis

Nasally inserted feeding tubes, 182
Needle-free connectors, 172; see also
    Sharps

Negative/positive air pressure rooms, 256–57, **258**, **259**
Neisseria meningitidis (Meningitis), 126–28, **259**
Norovirus, 132–37, **259**
Nurses, 8, 9–10, 89–90; *see also* Staffing procedures/precautions
Nutritional care, 177, 185; *see also* Milk preparation
  enteral feeding, 177–81
  nasally inserted feeding tubes, 182
  parenteral nutrition (PN), 184
  percutaneously inserted feeding tubes (PETS), 182–83

Operating theatre precautions, 222, 224–25; *see also* Peri-operative care

Pacemaker associated infection, 242–44
Paediatric settings, 197, 218
  milk preparation, 200–3
  playroom sessions, 199
  protective clothing, 198
  social contact, 198
  specific infections, **217**; *see also* Chickenpox; Measles; Mumps; RSV bronchiolitis
  toys, 198, 199–200
Palivizumab prophylaxis, 205
Parainfluenza, patient isolation requirements, **259**
Paramyxovirus infections, *see* Measles; Mumps
Parenteral nutrition (PN), 184
Parotitis, infectious (Mumps), 212–14, **259**
Parvovirus, **217**
Patient placement; *see also* Isolation; Ward transfers
  chickenpox, 208–9
  CJD/TSE, 123, 125
  Clostridium difficile infections, 109
  ESBL, infections 129
  glycopeptide resistant enterococci, **117**, 117–18
  isolated patients, 257, **259**
  measles infections, 214
  meningitis infections, 126
  MRSA infections, 98–99, 257, **259**, 269
  mumps infections, 212
  norovirus infections, 133, **259**
  respiratory syncytial virus infections, 204
  tuberculosis infections, **112**, 112–13, 115
PD (peritoneal dialysis), 249–50

Percutaneously inserted feeding tubes (PETS), 182–83
Peri-operative care, 220, 236
  anaesthesia, 220–22, **223**
  epidural catheters, 221–22
  gloving, 228–29
  gowning, 227–28
  operating theatre precautions, 222, 224–25
  post-anaesthesia care, 231
  prevention of surgical site infection, 229–31
  specific infections, 232–36, **235**
  surgical hand preparation, 226–27
Peripheral arterial catheters, 164–66
Peripheral venous cannulae (PVCs), 158–63
Peripherally inserted central venous catheters (PICCS), 169–70
Peritoneal dialysis (PD), 249–50
Personal protective equipment (PPE), 159; *see also* Protective clothing
Pertussis (Whooping cough), **217**, **259**, 271
PETS (percutaneously inserted feeding tubes), 182–83
Phagocytosis, 33
Phlebitis, 162–63, 164, 170
PICCS (Peripherally inserted central venous catheters), 169–70
Playroom sessions, 199
PN (parenteral nutrition), 184
Positive air pressure rooms, 256–57, **258**, **259**
Post-anaesthesia care, 231
PPE (personal protective equipment), 159; *see also* Protective clothing
Protective clothing
  aprons/gowns, 78–79
  chickenpox infections, 209
  CJD/TSE infections, 123
  Clostridium difficile infections, 107
  ESBL infections, 130
  eye protection, 81
  face-masks/respirators, 79–81, **81**
  gloves, 74–78, **75**, **76**, 157
  glycopeptide resistant enterococci infections, 118
  hepatitis infections, 92
  immunocompromised patients, 270
  measles infections, 215
  meningitis infections, 127
  MRSA infections, 101
  mumps infections, 212, 213
  nurse's uniforms, 89–90
  norovirus infections, 134
  paediatric settings, 198

respiratory syncytial virus infections, 205
tuberculosis infections, 113–14, 115
Protozoa, 22–23
Pseudomonas aeruginosa, **18**, 144, 221, 282

Quarantining surgical instruments, 236

Refrigerators, 202–3
Renal units, 246–50
Resistance, bacterial, 26–29, **28**, **29**, 97, 111; *see also* Chemotherapy; MRSA
Respirators, 79–81, **81**
Respiratory syncytial virus, 203–7, **259**
Ringworm, **217**
Risk assessment, 57–63, **61**, **64**
Rotavirus gastroenteritis, **217**, **259**
RSV (Respiratory syncytial virus) bronchiolitis, 203–7, **259**
Rubella (German measles), **259**, 271

Safety, environmental, 198–99
Salmonella spp., 3, 178, **259**, 271
Screening patients, for MRSA, 99–100
Sensitivity testing, micro-organisms, 24, **25**
Services, structure/function, 1, **6**, **9**, 11
  economic perspective, 5
  extent/prevalence of hospital acquired infections, 5–7, **7**
  governance processes, 10–11
  historical perspective, 1–3
  infection control nurses, 8, 9–10
  infection control structures/roles, 7–10
  legal infrastructure/codes of conduct, 3, 4, 5
Sharps (needles), 81–86, **83**, **85**
Shigella gastroenteritis, patient isolation requirements, **259**
Skin
  lesions, 58–59
  preparation, intravascular therapy, 157–58, 160
  role in immunity, 32
Slapped cheek (Parvovirus), **217**
Specialist care settings, 239, 251; *see also* Burns units; Cardiothoracic units; Intensive care units; Renal units
Specimen collection, 38, 55
  blood cultures, 47–50
  collection/storage/transport principles, 38–40
  faecal specimens, 46–47

meticillin resistant *Staphylococcus aureus* (MRSA), 51–52
respiratory syncytial virus, 205
sputum, 54–55
suction assisted nasal aspiration, 50–51, **51**
throat swabs, 52–54, **53**
tuberculosis, 115
urine specimens, 42–45
wound specimens, 40–42, 189–90
Spores, bacterial, 18
Sputum, specimen collection, 54–55
Staffing procedures/precautions, specific; *see also* Nurses
  chickenpox infections, 209
  ESBL infections, 130
  immunocompromised patients, 272
  measles infections, 214
  meningitis infections, 126
  mumps infections, 212
  norovirus infections, 133
  respiratory syncytial virus infections, 204–5
  tuberculosis infections, 113
Staphylococcus aureus, **18**, **24**; *see also* MRSA; VRSA
  antibiotic resistant strains, 1990s, 3
  burns units, 244, 245
  chemotherapy, 25
  epidural catheters, 221
  hand hygiene 68
  and immunocompromised patients, 268
  intravascular therapy, 156
  and urinary catheterisation, 144
  and VAP, 240
  wounds, 188
Sterilisation, 201, 275, 278–79; *see also* Decontamination
Stopcocks, 172
Storage principles, specimens, 38–40
Streptococcus spp. infections, **18**, 188, **259**
Suction assisted nasal aspiration, 50–51, **51**
Suctioning, 242
Surgical hand preparation, 226–27; *see also* Peri-operative care
Surveillance definitions, **6**
Swabs, 52–54, **53**,189–90

Throat swabs, 52–54, **53**
Tourniquets, 160
Toys, 198, 199–200
Tracheostomy management, 242
Transduction, bacterial, 27–29, **29**
Transfer, patient, *see* Ward transfers

Transformation, bacterial, 27, **28**
Transmissible spongiform encephalopathy, *see* TSE
Transmission routes, micro-organisms, 29–31, 97, 144
TSE (transmissible spongiform encephalopathy), 121–23, 234–36
  cleaning/decontamination procedures, 123–25, **125**
  definitions, **124**
  and endoscopy, 282
  infectivity and transmission risk, **123**
  patient discharge, 126
  quarantining instruments, 236
  surgical instrument management, **235**
Transporting specimens, 38–40
Tuberculosis, 110–12, 282
  cleaning procedures, 114–15
  and endoscopy, 282
  and HIV, 110
  patient discharge, 116
  patient placement/isolation, **112**, 112–13, 115, **259**
  peri-operative care, 232–33
  protective clothing, 113–14, 115
  specimens, 115
  treatment, 113

Urine specimens, 42–45
Urinary catheter care, 59, 140–41, 151
  biofilms, 143–4
  catheter associated urinary tract infection (CAUTI), 141
  catheterisation procedures, 145, 150–51
  evidence based guidelines, 145, **146–49**
  prevention principles, 141–42
  risk factors, 144–45
  routes of infection, 144
  suprapubic, 145

Vaccination, 36
Vancomycin resistant enterococci (VRE), 248, **259**
Vancomycin resistant *Staphylococcus aureus* (VRSA), 97; *see also* MRSA
VAP (Ventilator associated pneumonia), 240
Varicella zoster (Chickenpox), 207–11, **259**, 271
Vascular add-on devices, 171
vCJD, *see* TSE
Veins, inflammation (phlebitis), 162–63, 164, 170

Ventilator associated pneumonia (VAP), 240
Viral gastroenteritis, and peri-operative care, 233–34
Viruses, 18–21, **19**, **21**, 201, 246–48
Visitors, and specific infections
  chickenpox, 211
  CJD/TSE, 125
  Clostridium difficile, 109
  ESBL infections, 132
  glycopeptide resistant enterococci, 120
  immunocompromised patients, 271
  measles, 216
  meningitis, 128
  MRSA, 104
  mumps, 213–14
  norovirus, 135
  respiratory syncytial virus, 207
  tuberculosis, 115

Ward transfers, and specific infections
  chickenpox, 210
  ESBL infections, 131
  isolated patients, 263
  measles, 215–16
  meningitis, 128
  MRSA, 104
  mumps, 213
  respiratory syncytial virus, 206–7
Waste handling, 86–87
  chickenpox, 210
  CJD/TSE, 125
  Clostridium difficile, 108
  ESBL infections, 131
  glycopeptide resistant enterococci, 119
  isolated patients, 262
  measles, 215
  meningitis, 127
  MRSA, 103
  mumps, 212
  norovirus, 134
  respiratory syncytial virus, 206
  tuberculosis, 114
Water for drinking, and immunocompromised patients 270
Whooping cough, (Pertussis), **217**, **259**, 271
Wound management, 187–88, 194–95
  dressing techniques, 190–93
  identifying infection, 189–90
  infection prevention/management, 190, 194
  sampling for infection, 40–42, 189–90